Contents

Acknowledgements

This book is dedicated to Hanne Marquardt, Anthony Porter and Kristine Walker, who are all outstanding reflexologists in their own field, and whose inspiration over the years has encouraged me to explore my own discoveries in reflexology.

My appreciation and thanks goes to all my wonderful VRT tutors. To Anna Crago and all at Piatkus Books, and to my agent Michael Alcock for their patience and encouragement. To Lesley Wakerley for the excellent illustrations. To my friends and colleagues for their invaluable input: Mary Atkinson, Carol Clark, Denise Hopley, Nick Hounsfield, Pauline Noakes, Jean Roberts and Christina Shewell. To Mr Lindsay McMillan, FRCOG, for his exceptional skills as a surgeon and for his openness in researching both the conventional and complementary aspects of medicine. To Gerald Lee, Director, and all the staff and residents at the St Monica Trust, Bristol, for their interest in and cooperation with my work. To Hedwige Dirkx, Maggie Lansdown and Janet Woodward for their great help with the illustrations. To Esther Forte and Margaret Kingwell for their office support. To my clients and VRT practitioners. Thanks also to my dear parents, brothers and sister. Finally, a special mention for Adam and Alice with grateful loving thanks for being there.

About the Author

Lynne Booth BA (Hons), BRCP, MIIR (regd), ART (Hons), MAR was trained at the International Institute of Reflexology in London. She runs a private practice and nursing home clinic in Bristol, England and has used reflexology in a hospital setting. In 1998 ART (Advanced Reflexology Training) awarded her an honorary fellowship for services to reflexology. She lectures in Britain and internationally, has spoken at NHS seminars for the medical profession and runs professional training courses for reflexologists in VRT. She is the author of *Vertical Reflexology*.

Vertical Reflexology For Hands

A revolutionary five-minute technique
to transform your health

Lynne Booth

PIATKUS

VRT does not replace normal allopathic and medical treatment. It is a means of supporting and complementing such medical treatment. If you have any acute or chronic disease you should seek medical attention from a qualified medical doctor. The author and publisher accept no liability for damage of any nature resulting directly or indirectly from the application or use of information in this book.

First published in 2003 by
Judy Piatkus (Publishers) Limited
5 Windmill Street
London W1T 2JA
e-mail: info@piatkus.co.uk

VRT
THE BOOTH METHOD

For the latest news and information on all our titles, visit our website at www.piatkus.co.uk

A catalogue record for this book is available from the British Library

ISBN 0 7499 2319 9

Edited by Sandra Rigby
Text design by Jerry Goldie
Illustrated by Lesley Wakerley

This book has been printed on paper manufactured
with respect for the environment using wood from
managed sustainable resources

Printed and bound in Great Britain by
Butler & Tanner Ltd, Frome, Somerset

Foreword

Throughout my years involved with training people in reflexology I have worked with some very talented and dedicated reflexologists. Lynne Booth is one whose natural talent and enthusiasm makes her shine.

After qualifying with the International Institute of Reflexology, Lynne then studied ART (Advanced Reflexology Training). Her passion and enthusiasm for the techniques quickly made her a first-class practitioner with a large following of highly satisfied patients. In 1998 she was awarded an ART honorary fellowship.

When practising reflexology our main aim is to constantly explore new avenues and techniques that will benefit our patients. Lynne has certainly achieved that goal with VRT. What she has discovered is a major contribution to, if not a quantum leap in, the great therapeutic benefits that VRT bestows. Vertical Reflexology for Hands takes us up another rung in the ladder of further understanding in reflexology.

A VRT hand treatment is highly effective, quick and economical to both the patient and the practitioner. Lynne Booth's book is a gem. Buy it, try it, learn it!

Anthony J Porter
Founder/Director, Advanced Reflexology Training

Anthony Porter began his career in massage and bodywork and has been a reflexologist for 30 years. He was British and European Director of the International Institute of Reflexology and spent many years lecturing internationally with the president, Dwight Byers. In 1984 he formed ART (Advanced Reflexology Training) to provide post-graduate clinical training for reflexologists. He has published a reflexology textbook and practises in a London clinic specialising in the treatment of gynaecological and hormonal conditions.

To Hanne Marquardt, Anthony Porter and Kristine Walker

Introduction

Hands are one of the most familiar and important parts of our bodies. They help us to feed and clothe ourselves, they protect us, they allow us to communicate with others, and they can also help us to heal. In this book you will learn how to use Vertical Reflex Therapy (VRT) for hands to heal both other people and yourself.

VRT is a fast and effective form of reflexology that is applied to the hands and feet when they are weight-bearing, that is, when your palms are resting on a flat surface or you are standing on your feet. VRT techniques produce extraordinary results that enable the body to help itself to heal. In addition to hand VRT techniques, this book introduces nail-working and unique nail-on-nail techniques. These allow the therapist to work all the zones in the body through a grid system in the nails. These techniques work in a very powerful way when connected with specific reflexes and are described in detail in Chapter 5.

Reflexology stimulates tiny reflex points on the hands or feet that together form a mini-map of the body. Many minute reflexes, or stimulation points, cover the entire hand, and every part of the hand relates to a particular part of the body. Working the hands with the aid of VRT charts is rather like having access to a junction box that needs tuning and maintaining to help keep the body in a healthy condition. For example, by pressing the tip and base of your thumb you can often help get rid of a headache, and anyone feeling nervous before an interview or exam can discreetly press a part of their hand below the thumb that is connected to the adrenal reflex area. This should calm the rush of adrenalin and help to balance the body. You can also discreetly stimulate your hands to ease indigestion or release a stiff neck, and there are ways to stop a child or adult feeling travel-sick. You'll learn all these techniques, and much more, in this book.

VRT techniques offer you control over your health in a gentle and non-invasive way. Reflexology aims to bring about balance or homeostasis to the body so, for example, if the adrenal glands are excreting too much adrenalin then the aim is to reduce that. Conversely, if you felt lethargic and worked the same pressure points, they would be stimulated to revitalise a tired body.

Many of the techniques in this book have been developed from VRT for the feet, which I developed over the last decade, and which were described in my previous book, *Vertical Reflexology*. This book explains the many benefits of working the hands and the results are equally good, if not better in some cases, than those gained from working the feet. In fact, the hands are often a more popular choice for VRT treatment as they are more accessible than the feet, making it much easier to carry out self help or discreet treatments on others.

The success of my first book, *Vertical Reflexology*, has helped me to spread the word that reflexology really is accessible to everyone, whether you are a professional reflexologist, a complementary therapist, or just an interested reader who would like to learn how to treat yourself, your family and your friends. VRT is very simple to apply and the body responds readily even to the amateur touch.

VRT is a relatively new development in complementary care – I discovered and developed it during the mid-1990s. For the past nine years I have run a weekly reflexology clinic at one of the largest residential care homes in the UK, the St Monica Trust in Bristol. This charitable trust cares for 200 elderly people, offering them sheltered housing as well as 24-hour nursing care. It has pioneered an innovative range of health care and opportunities for its residents.

While working at the trust as a conventional reflexologist, I found that I could not always access the soles of the feet of wheelchair-bound residents because of their pain, heavily ulcerated legs or lack of mobility. This led me to experiment with working the dorsum (top) of a client's weight-bearing foot or hand as they sat in their wheelchair, and I found that I could obtain excellent results.

I began to work on the tops of the feet much more, and found that people appeared to be getting better more quickly than I would have expected with conventional reflexology. Skeletal problems responded most quickly, but all ailments, including intractable chronic problems such as constipation and blocked sinuses, responded well.

Like many discoveries, the most significant move in the development of VRT came about due to a combination of intuition, research and practical application to solve an immediate problem. I gave first aid to an elderly female resident in the home. Her hip and leg had been injured in a recent accident and she was shuffling along on a Zimmer frame. I had to think laterally to overcome a difficult situation: gentle, immediate therapy was required. I knelt down and worked her feet for a few seconds while she was in the standing position. Within half an hour of my treatment she felt pain, tingling and then relief in her hip, and by the following day she was almost pain free and could raise her leg higher than she had been able to do before the accident. I immediately realised that it was full weight-bearing pressure that caused the reflexes to trigger such a powerful, and often immediate, response, and from then on developed specific techniques for the weight-bearing hands and feet.

The fact that these chronically sick residents responded so positively to weight-bearing hand and foot reflexology convinced me that these gentle skills could be used to help heal everyone from the tiniest baby to an octogenarian. I shared my findings with many reflexologist colleagues who in turn shared them with others, all of whom achieved similar results to mine as soon as they applied what began to be known in reflexology circles as the Booth Method.

Vertical reflexology thus became totally integrated into my practice and I treated each client with a few minutes of hand or foot VRT at every treatment. In 1997 I decided to undertake a small, medically approved trial at the St Monica Trust to test the efficacy of VRT. During the seven-week trial we saw chronically ill people with multiple health problems respond both physically and emotionally to the short, non-invasive vertical reflexology treatments. The trial, despite its small scale, was an important landmark in the research and development of VRT, as it demonstrated the body's innate ability to self-heal when given the correct impetus. After seven weeks over 60 per cent of the client group showed a measurable improvement, and this improvement had been maintained two months later when I published a paper on the trial.

Many of the case study examples in this book come from VRT practitioners who have seen a wide range of positive results in their clients after they have received VRT on their hands or feet. The hands and feet contain the same number of reflexes and both offer a window into the body, enabling any condition to be treated in a holistic way.

Vertical Reflexology for Hands is very much a 'hands-on' book and will teach you the techniques that have proved so effective for me and my colleagues. One of the benefits of the treatments you will learn is that they are short – a maximum of five minutes – but they can also be included in a full 30- to 35-minute hand reflexology treatment. You will not only learn how to treat the hands of family, friends and clients, but will also discover very effective self-help techniques.

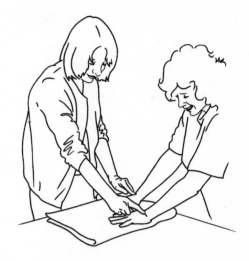

Weight-bearing hand reflexology

The first half of this book teaches the various techniques, both basic and advanced, and explains how to find the necessary pressure points on the hands. The second half of the book is a brief survey of each system of the body, covering:

- How VRT can help each system, and general tips for useful techniques.
- An example of a typical ailment for each system – for instance earache, stress, Irritable Bowel Syndrome, angina and stroke.
- A specific treatment for that particular ailment using nail reflexes.

- Self-help techniques.
- Optional complementary help which may benefit those with ailments falling into this category.

Reflexology and VRT are highly effective in relieving stress, improving circulation and stimulating the body to help itself. It is estimated that over 75 per cent of illnesses are stress-related – as the body's defence system becomes weakened when it exists in a constant state of tension, we become much more vulnerable to illness and disease. We often wring or grip our hands when stressed. How much better to practise self-help VRT and gently press the hands in a directed fashion to rid ourselves of tension. Hand VRT, even if only applied for five minutes twice a week, is a way of giving our bodies a regular service. Good health is the most valuable possession we have, as it helps us to live life to the full, to work and contribute to the good of others and fulfil loving relationships.

Be kind to your body, it is the only place you live.

Part 1

Vertical Reflex Therapy hand techniques

Chapter 1

Understanding hand reflexology

The origins of the ancient healing science of reflexology go back 5,000 years to China, India and Egypt. Similar techniques were also used by the Native Americans and the Mayans in South America 1,500 years ago. Forms of reflexology reached Europe in the Dark Ages after Marco Polo opened up the silk routes in the thirteenth century, and were used by both peasants and the aristocracy as a pressure-point therapy on the hands and feet. However, it was not until the 1930s that an American physiotherapist called Eunice Ingham developed the zone and pressure-point therapy that is reflexology as we know it today. Ingham was assistant to Dr Joe Shelby Riley, a physician, who wrote four books on Zone Therapy and extensively researched and taught its role in pain control.

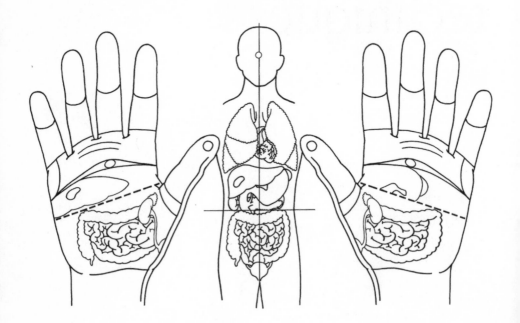

Each hand mirrors half of the body

Zone Therapy forms the basis of hand and foot reflexology. An American ear, nose and throat surgeon, Dr William Fitzgerald (1872–1942), carried the existing theory of reflexology further and divided the body into ten vertical zones – five on the left-hand side of the body, and five on the right. Each zone relates to all parts of the body within its boundaries. The hands and feet mirror these zones, and can be manipulated to affect corresponding parts of the body via energetic impulses which are connected to organs, glands and skeletal systems within the zones. The head area is represented in the fingers or toes, the chest area on the balls of the hands or feet, the abdominal area on the lower palm or plantar, and the hip, pelvic and knee areas in the regions of the wrist and ankles. The diagram opposite shows the areas of the hand that correspond to the different parts of the body, while the diagram below shows the ten energy zones reflected in the hands.

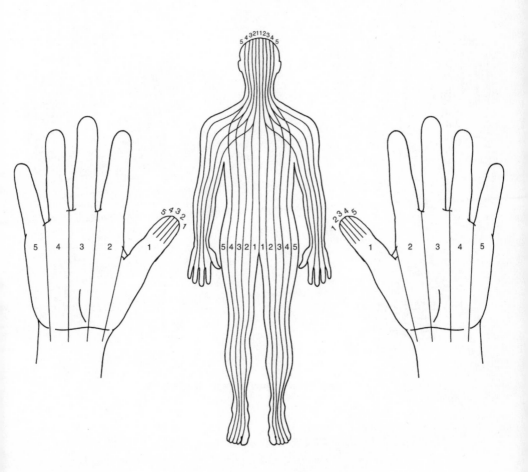

The ten reflexology zones of the body

The basic premise of reflexology is that tension or disease in the body creates an imbalance in the body's life force, and this is manifested in tender reflexes in the hands and feet. Sometimes sensitive reflexes can indicate that an energetic impulse from a reflex to a corresponding organ or body part is blocked or congested. Gentle stimulation of a particular reflex can cause the congested area to clear, thus allowing an acceleration of repair work and healing to naturally occur in the body. VRT helps to sensitise the reflexes and magnify this response not only by clearing a pathway for the reflex but also by opening up a zone (which is one-tenth of the body). It's rather like flushing out a blocked pipe.

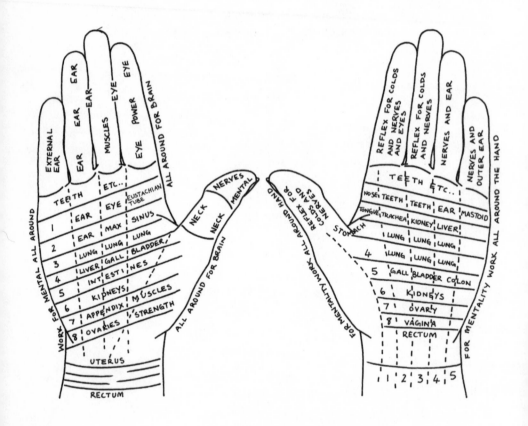

An early hand chart by Dr Joe Shelby Riley

Reflexologists do not prescribe, diagnose or treat specific illnesses; instead they work on the body to help to stimulate and balance its own healing response. Therapists are taught to work various reflexes to help certain conditions and to encourage the body to heal itself.

While the benefits of conventional reflexology are well known, working the
weight-bearing hands – especially VRT
nail-working – offers new and exciting
possibilities for therapists. The charts,
methods and techniques described in this
book can be used by a variety of people,
both professional and non-professional.
They are also very effective as self-help
treatments. As no manipulation or invasion
of the body (such as the insertion of
needles) takes place in reflexology it is the
ideal therapy to use, in its most basic form,
on family or friends or as self-help. VRT
makes the body exceptionally receptive to
gentle pressure on the reflexes, and many
minor ailments can be helped or cured by
an amateur touch as long as the contraindications and guidelines listed on pages
8–9 are followed.

Guidelines for reflexologists

- Reflexologists do not diagnose, prescribe or treat specific conditions separately. They work in a non-invasive way to trigger the body's own healing response.

- Reflexologists are trained to specifically work the systems of the body on the hands and feet.

- VRT and reflexology can be used independently but they also complement other natural therapies and conventional medication.

- Reflexology is preventative as well as curative. Babies and geriatrics, the sick and the healthy can all respond to this healing touch.

The benefits of hand reflexology

Reflexology has always been an attractive therapy for many people as the feet
are easily accessible for treatment and there is no need to undress. Hand reflexology takes the accessibility of reflexology one step further as our hands are
almost always uncovered and available for touch. The most passive or comatose

CASE STUDY

Joyce was an active pensioner who had enjoyed playing tennis since she was
eleven. After a mastectomy, she was offered reflexology by her hospital and followed up her introductory treatments with some VRT and conventional treatment. Her intention was to play tennis again as soon as possible, and my main
aim was to help accelerate the healing of the scar tissue due to the removal of
the lymph glands under the arm. After four treatments she could raise her arm
and stretch it without feeling a painful pull under the arm. Three months later
she resumed playing tennis again. I also taught Joyce self-help VRT on her hands
to aid her recovery in between treatments.

CASE STUDY

In a conventional reflexology trial on patients with dysmenorrhea (severe period pain) at Whipps Cross Hospital in London, consultant gynaecological surgeon, Mr Lindsay McMillan describes how his year-long trial was not completed as 'it became blatantly obvious that reflexology was far superior to the then current surgical treatment for severe dysmenorrhea and I felt that it was unethical for me to continue the trial'.

Mr McMillan worked closely throughout the trial with a reflexologist, Anthony Porter. Mr McMillan outlines the aim of the trial and the results below.

'In 1994 I took a number of young women who all suffered refractory dysmenorrhea and complained of very severe pain at the time of their periods. Many of the women would be hospitalised due to their extreme discomfort. All these patients had had conventional treatment such as combined oral contraceptives, non-steroidal anti-inflammatories and analgesia at the time of their periods with little or no effect on their pain.

At that time there was a theory that if one transected the nerve fibres that run on the medial aspect of both uterosacral ligaments this would cure the pain experienced at the time of the period, but I had serious doubts from personal experience.

Knowing Anthony Porter could often alleviate dysmenorrhea with reflexology, we set up a trial which involved me choosing the patients and randomly selecting them for either surgery or a course of reflexology.

In the first group of patients – those selected for surgery – other pathology such as endometriosis was excluded from their pelvis. If there was no obvious evidence of other pathology, surgery was carried out.

The course of reflexology we set out for the second group of patients was to have a session of reflexology once a week for the four weeks leading up to their menstrual bleed. In the second month, they would have two treatments in the two weeks prior to their menses. In the third month, there would be two weekly treatments in the two weeks prior to their menses, and thereafter a single treatment in the week before the onset of their menses.

By the end of nine to ten months, when we began to correlate the figures, it became obvious that Anthony's success in alleviating severe dysmenorrhea in these women was in the region of 85–90 per cent, whereas in surgical treatment it was probably less than half that figure.

It was at this point that I made the difficult decision that I could not submit women for a potentially dangerous procedure under general anaesthesia when it seemed the results were so unfavourable compared to reflexology.'

hospital patient will usually have a hand available to be held and, if appropriate, treated. Working the hands can be extremely discreet and I have quietly worked the hands of a child who felt car-sick while travelling, or held a friend's hand in the theatre and worked the stomach reflex to ease a bout of indigestion. I teach asthmatic children to press their hand on a desk and work the bronchial reflexes gently to stop them wheezing. When nervous, especially before an interview or exam, you can work the adrenal gland reflex on the fleshy thenar muscle on your hand to help calm yourself down.

It appears that as soon as the hand becomes weight-bearing, even partially when pressed against one's leg, the power is turned up as far as the therapeutic response is concerned, and the body appears to be able to react more quickly. It is not always possible to work on a fully weight-bearing hand if someone is bedridden, for example, but some of the basic hand reflexology techniques in Chapter 3 can be adapted so that pressure can be applied to a hand that is pressing downwards onto a small bedside table.

VRT also has many benefits for the practitioner both from a postural aspect and from the expansion of the ways in which the hands are physically used. Standard reflexology requires the therapist to sit at the end of a couch or reclining chair for 30 to 60 minutes, barely changing position, with their forefinger and thumb precisely and repetitively working all the reflexes on the hands and feet. The VRT practitioner has a whole new arena of movement: if the feet are worked while the client is standing the therapist will be kneeling and moving on the floor for a few minutes, and various techniques allow the reflexologist to move, stand or walk about during a conventional hand or foot treatment. The various uses of knuckles within VRT gives the digits a rest and utilises another part of the hands.

The benefits of hand VRT
● Improved circulation.
● Stimulation of the immune system.
● Release of tension.
● Powerful simple self-help methods.
● Possible increase in mobility and decrease in pain.
● Relaxing non-invasive techniques.

Who can be safely treated?

Most people, from tiny babies to the very elderly, can benefit from reflexology. The US-based International Institute of Reflexology suggests that no one need be excluded, whereas some schools of reflexology give students a long list of contraindications. The professional opinions and decisions of individual bodies should be respected and I would advise reflexologists to follow their own training and only treat conditions with which they feel comfortable.

One of the prime reasons for administering reflexology is to help the

PRACTITIONER'S CASE STUDY

Condition: Painful elbow.

Client: Female. **Aged:** 35.

Duration of illness: Two to three years.

No. of VRT treatments: Five.

Aim of treatment: To relieve pain in elbow.

Result: Immediate relief after first session. Played squash before second session and felt fine. Played squash after third session and felt pain. After third VRT treatment she had no further pain.

Practitioner's comments: The symptoms of tennis elbow seem to return after the first and second treatments but are gone by the third or fourth. This also appears to be the case for various other joint problems.

Author's comment: Excellent results can be obtained on orthopaedic problems. VRT was discovered through treating such conditions and they seem to respond more quickly than others.

circulation of lymph to cleanse and boost the immune system. If we work the body in this way, by stimulating the thymus and lymphatic reflexes as well as all organs and glands, we are helping to fight disease, whether it is a mild infection or a serious condition. The stimulation of the immune and lymph systems will help to detoxify the body whether the client is suffering from cancer or sinusitis. It will not spread infection – it will fight it. That's why, in my personal experience, I have found very few conditions that do not respond favourably to reflexology.

However, if you are not a qualified reflexologist you should avoid treating people with any of the conditions listed below. Professional training and knowledge of anatomy and physiology are required to treat them properly.

Contraindications

- **Deep Vein Thrombosis (DVT)** To be avoided totally except by professional therapists after the recovery period. Professional reflexologists often work the lower arm referral area, which means that the leg or foot of a DVT sufferer need not be touched.

- **Varicose veins** Treat the person but do not work directly on the veins. Using hand VRT overcomes this problem.

- **Epilepsy** Some professional reflexologists have achieved good results with epileptic conditions but unless you are fully qualified and have worked with or experienced treatment of a person with epilepsy previously, do not treat.

- **Pregnancy** You can work the hands very gently but avoid the reproductive reflexes in the first four months.

- **Heart problems** Work the hands very gently and brush over the heart reflex so it is touched but not overworked. The new helper heart/diaphragm reflexes on the wrist will enable the heart to be stimulated indirectly but effectively. Always work the sigmoid colon reflex gently when treating heart conditions, as there appears to be a correlation between these two reflexes in the same zone.

Key points to remember

- Never diagnose an illness, override or ignore medical advice or advise anyone to stop taking medication unless this has been authorised by a doctor.

- Do not promise to cure specific ailments or guarantee a cure and beware of any therapist who does so. It is not only unethical to do so, but also highly unlikely that the desired results will be achieved.

- When seeking a complementary practitioner, always check their credentials thoroughly and ask if they are insured and a member of a professional body.

- Never underestimate the body's capacity to help heal itself.

- Complementary medicine by definition indicates that natural and allopathic therapies can work successfully together. It is helpful if the client lets their doctor know they are receiving VRT and reflexology.

- Gritty or tender reflexes do not always indicate a major health problem. Tender reflexes can also indicate vitality!

Chapter 2

Conventional hand reflexology techniques

This section introduces you to the traditional reflexology finger and thumb techniques that can be used on the hands and feet. You will also learn the basic moves for conventional hand reflexology on the passive hands. Refer to the Glossary (page 186) for any unfamiliar terms.

Most reflexology techniques are best practised on your own hands and arms first, to feel the pressure and sensation they achieve. The thumb is used extensively in reflexology but it is the sides of the thumbs that are used, not the tips or the nail itself, except with the unique VRT nail-working taught in Chapter 5. A gentle pressure from all your nails as you curl your fingers into the palm reflexes is permissible. It is very helpful to practise on a model of a hand. You can buy these from your local joke shop, or from a supplier of latex hands.

Strengthening your hands

You may find that your hands, fingers and thumbs will feel very stiff or sore in the early days of practising reflexology. At first, the precise movements required for this therapeutic technique can leave the hands aching as they will have been using some tiny, little used muscles and joints in repetitive movements.

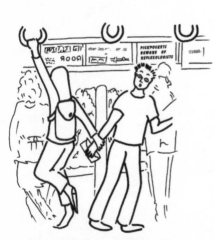

Pickpockets beware of reflexologists!
Courtesy Kristine Walker

It is important for every therapist to look after and exercise their hands, as they are our means of helping others and earning a living. Many reflexologists keep their hands healthy by exercising with purpose-built sprung grippers, which can be squeezed repeatedly to build up muscular strength. The tendons in the hands can easily become strained and it is worth paying attention to your body's posture and the angle of your hands when you work.

I realised how strong my small hands had become through reflexology when a pickpocket on an Amsterdam tram tried to steal my purse from my backpack. I reached up and gripped his hand tightly until he let go of the purse and ran off.

Preparing the hands for reflexology

Before you begin any hand reflexology session, take a moment to familiarise yourself with your client's hands. Remember that the hands are thinner and less firm in texture than the feet and must be worked in a very sensitive and gentle manner. Extra-firm pressure will not achieve extra healing results – only discomfort and unwillingness on the part of the client to return.

Feel and familiarise yourself with the five longest bones of the hands, the metacarpals. When you first hold a person's hands, observe the general feel, texture and condition of the nails. Look at the colour of the skin. Is it patchy, mottled, fleshy or dry and flaky? Are the nails brittle? These features can sometimes indicate poor circulation or a nutritional deficiency. Sometimes there will be rough, dry patches on the skin or calluses on the balls of the hands (or feet) and this often indicates a lung/chest weakness as the thickened skin appears to be directly situated on the reflex. When a client has a cluster of warts on their hands then work that area on the feet instead. Keep tea tree oil available during treatments to apply with a swab of cotton wool to any verruca, warts or fungal areas on the hands or feet, or cover with a plaster.

Before treating a client, you will need to wash your hands or clean them with an antiseptic wipe. You may choose to use some non-oily cream to help you work into a reflex, although you will only need a small amount. Many reflexologists prefer to only work with a dry hand and use no cream or just a little cornstarch.

Looking after the hands

- Keep your hands clean, and dry them well after washing.
- Keep the nails short and filed.
- Both men and women should regularly use a gentle hand cream to protect and moisturise the skin.
- Wear rubber or surgical gloves when using any cleaners – even mild household detergents can cause dryness and rashes.
- When gardening wear leather or cloth gloves.
- Occasionally, before bed, soak your hands in warm water for up to five minutes and rub them with a deeply penetrating, oil-based cream or calendula (marigold) oil. Wear cloth gloves in bed at night to avoid marking the sheets. Calendula oil is especially helpful if the hands are chapped, and can be used regularly for a week or two if this is the case.
- In the winter wear warm gloves to protect your hands.

Before you begin a session you will also need to check that you have the basic equipment necessary. You will need one or two hard, upright chairs, or a couch or recliner chair; a small table (if using chairs); pillow(s) or cushions(s) to rest the hands/elbows; soft terry-towels and mild antiseptic wipes.

Positions for treating the client

Many hand reflexologists have two upright chairs facing each other across a small table and the client rests their elbows on a cushion or towel placed on the table. Otherwise, sit facing each other on upright chairs with cushion(s) placed on the client's lap as shown. Ensure that your arms are at the correct angle so you do not strain your hands.

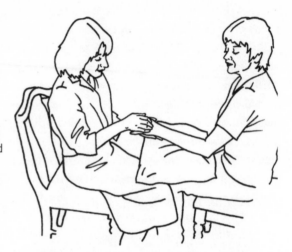

Client and therapist using cushion for support

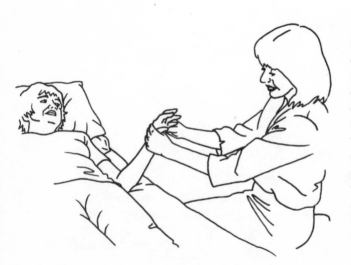

If you work with a couch or reclining chair you will need to place your own chair alongside the couch. Couches are usually fairly high and you may need to add a cushion to your chair to gain height. Start by wiping their hands with an antiseptic wipe before introducing some relaxation techniques.

Using a couch or reclining chair

Position of the client's passive hands

The position of the client's passive (that is, non-weight-bearing) hands is important. The client should rest on their elbows and hold their arms loose, but upright, so that their relaxed hands can be worked from different angles. The client's hands can be firmly worked using your thumb, second and third fingers for best results. Approach the palm from behind and gently press your nails into their palm reflexes in a rolling movement. This will not hurt and stimulates the reflexes.

Basic relaxation techniques

Now you are ready to begin with some general relaxation techniques. The following techniques are to be used when a person is sitting or lying down and resting their elbows on a cushion. They can be introduced at the beginning of a conventional reflexology treatment. They can also be used in conjunction with a combined VRT/standard reflexology session, or with Diaphragm Rocking (see page 52) in between VRT treatments. Using the relaxation techniques will make the entire body more responsive to reflexology.

Loosening the wrists

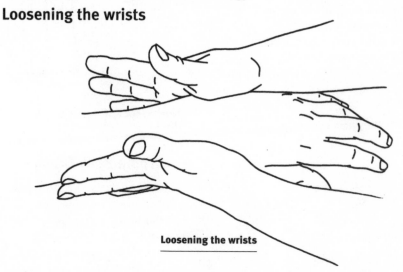

Loosening the wrists

Cup the heel of your palms on either side of the wrist-bones and press firmly so the hand is secure. Shake the client's wrist and hand by evenly moving your own hands up and down the sides of their hand in opposite directions. As your right hand moves forwards, your left hand should slide backwards a little, and then the movement is reversed. Allow your fingers and upper hand to become more flexible so that they gently slap the sides of the hands. Repeat on the other hand. This is excellent for improving circulation and preventing cold or 'dead' fingers, especially in the winter.

Twisting the spinal reflexes

Place both hands, side by side, over the top of the right hand you are working, and with your fingers pointing to the outside or lateral edge of the hand. Your forefingers will be touching as you grip the hand. Your two thumbs touch the palm of the client's hand and the webbing of your thumb is pressed firmly against the spinal reflexes on the inside or medial edge of the hand. Do not move the hand closest to the client's wrist but simply use it to grip their hand firmly. Your other hand grips and turns their hand in a rotating movement backwards and forwards in a pleasant stretching sensation. Then slide both hands about an inch towards the fingers and repeat the movements. Continue to inch up the hand until the edge of your hand (little finger) covers the client's fingers. Repeat on the left hand.

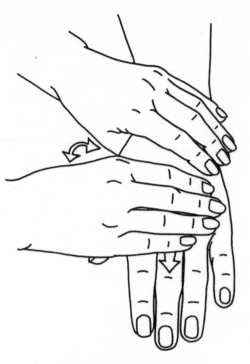

Twisting the spinal reflexes

Whole body brush

Whole Body Brush

Place your client's hand in your hands with your fingertips touching their wrist bracelet and pointing in the direction of their arms. Press your eight fingers gently but firmly on the skin. Your thumbs rest on the hand. Then inch both hands simultaneously towards you in tiny little movements. The whole movement should flow from the wrists to the fingertips, tenderly but firmly enough for the client to be aware of the intermittent pressure. The movements are made three times starting from the client's wrists on each hand. The first pass along the hand is firm and stimulating and the second should be lighter and allow your fingers to slide more. The third pass should consist of a gentle brushing, soothing movement with your fingertips. Repeat on the left hand.

Key hand movements

Now that you have learnt some basic relaxation techniques, it's time to familiarise yourself with the key practical hand movements used in hand reflexology.

Holding the hand

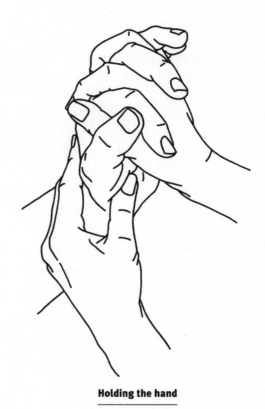

- Hold the client's right hand with your left hand, and use your right hand to work the reflexes. In turn, hold their left hand with your right hand, using your left as the working hand. It is easier to work their hand if their elbow is placed on a pillow and their hand is in an upright position. It is also acceptable to work their hand as it rests on the pillow, which can be on a lap or a small, low table.

- Keep their right hand palm upwards and link the fingers of your left hand through theirs. Your thumb will be placed between their thumb and index finger. You can then support and turn their hand as you work specific reflexes with your right hand.

Holding the hand

Thumb pressure walking

- Practise on yourself by placing your left hand, palm downwards, on a table. Turn your thumb slightly on its side so that the outer edge is touching the table. With the working right hand bend the thumb at the first joint, about 45 degrees, nearest the nail. If the thumb is straight or bent on the second joint it will cause strain and will not be at the correct angle to work the reflexes.

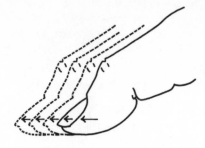

Thumb pressure walking

- Inch your thumb along in tiny movements as if you are pressing on a series of pinpoints. Try the same movements on your other hand and this time press firmly into your skin so that you are aware of different sensations as you work.

- Become aware of the fleshy and bony parts of your hands, of rough skin, and whether the hand feels warm or cool, and check if any parts of your hand feel tender to the touch.

Your aim is to develop a firm, even pressure and sensitivity to changes in the feel of the hands, which could indicate that a particular reflex needs stimulating.

Finger pressure walking

The same principles and techniques also apply to the finger. The corner lateral edge of the index finger is used and the first joint only is bent at 45 degrees as it works across the hand.

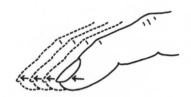

Finger pressure walking

- Tender reflexes need to be approached from several angles to make sure all the areas have been covered. Make sure that your body as well as your hands and fingers are at the most comfortable angle to avoid strain.

- Use three or four fingers (as described in the Whole Body Brush, page 14), to cover a greater area more quickly. Place the emphasis on the fingertips pressing and brushing the skin.

- Sometimes a reflex can feel sore, tender or gritty to the touch. The side of your finger can work into these points from different angles and often achieves a threefold effect of dispersing the granulation, easing a tender reflex and improving a specific condition in the body.

The use of knuckles in reflexology

Knuckles are not traditionally used in reflexology but practitioners such as Anthony Porter of Advanced Reflexology Training have developed and taught very powerful techniques using knuckles. The hip, pelvic and knee reflexes respond particularly well to these techniques, and repetitive strain problems are less likely if a greater variety of techniques is used.

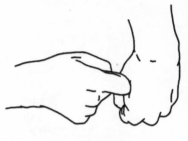

A knuckle technique

Knuckle-working method

Orthopaedic problems sometimes respond almost instantly when a knuckle gently works the hip, knee and pelvic reflexes around the wrists. You may want to use a small amount of cream. To practise, apply the following moves.

- Bend all your fingers at the second joint to form a knuckle.

- Tuck your thumb under your fingers loosely or leave it naturally out-stretched.

- Raise the knuckle of your index finger slightly and practise on your other hand by pressing and twisting it over a small area using the side of your knuckle.

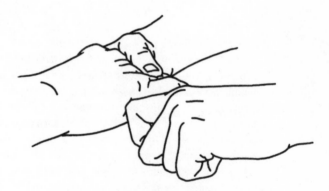

Using knuckle on the lateral dorsal spine reflex

Method – tip of knuckle

- Press the reflex with your knuckle and slightly rock your hands backwards and forwards from the wrist.

- Work the client's hand, feeling your knuckle stretch across the surface as it slides up and down the palm or dorsum (top of the hand).

- Return to the same point and repeat the pressing and sliding motion two or three times as you work a specific reflex.

- Use just enough lubrication to allow the knuckle to slide slowly backwards and forwards over the reflexes.

First steps towards VRT nail-working

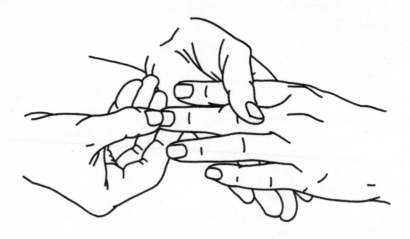

First steps towards nail-working

- Take the client's left hand in your left hand and turn it so it is facing palm downwards. Place your four fingers underneath the medial (inside) edge of their hand and put your thumb-tip at wrist level in zone 1 (see page 47) in alignment with the thumb. Now pinch down the hand in a line along the first metacarpal (one of the principal bones in the hand – see page 46) and continue down the thumb in small bites until the tip of your thumb-pad touches their thumbnail. Arch your thumb and place the tip of your thumbnail at the base of their thumbnail and edge your thumbnail along the centre of the nail to the tip. It is essential that you lightly and repeatedly touch your nail on the client's nail while moving the pad of your forefinger along the client's thumb until you reach the tip of their nail.

- Return to the wrist and work zones 2 and 3 (see page 47). Take your right hand and, holding their same hand, work zone 4 up from the wrist, and then the little finger. Again use your thumb to work nail-on-nail. Repeat on the right hand. This is a profound and calming treatment and gently stimulates the various reflexes under the nails. Full details of VRT nail-working are in Chapter 5.

With the basic reflexology moves now covered, you are ready to move on to a conventional hand reflexology treatment.

> **PRACTITIONER'S CASE STUDY**
>
> **Condition:** Cancer of the sigmoid colon.
>
> **Client:** Female. **Aged:** 63.
>
> **Duration of illness:** One year.
>
> **Aim of treatment:** To help the original medical diagnosis of angina.
>
> **Result:** The reflexes indicated that the problem was not with the heart but was emanating from the bowel.
>
> **Practitioner's comments:** The sigmoid colon was found to be extremely tender. Haemorrhoids (piles) were then suggested when blood appeared in the client's stools. Bowel cancer was eventually diagnosed and treated, all the angina symptoms disappeared, and the client's strong heart medication was discontinued.
>
> **Author's comment:** It has been suggested that the sigmoid colon should be worked in cases of heart problems rather than a concentration on the heart reflex as both are in the same zone. I always bear this point in mind although I am careful not to make a diagnosis when working the sigmoid colon to strengthen the heart reflex. In this case the therapist used lateral thinking and correctly deduced that the angina-like symptoms were caused by a chronic bowel condition.

Conventional hand reflexology techniques

These techniques will enable you to give a conventional hand reflexology treatment that will treat the body in an holistic manner. The hand charts on pages 25–6 will help you to identify areas of congestion in the body. Often major or minor imbalances in the body will manifest themselves in a physical change to the reflexes. The client may report a bruised, tender or pricking sensation and the therapist may be aware of a granular, puffy or firmer feel to the reflexes.

Once you have mastered a general treatment on the passive hands you will be able to combine this with the basic hand VRT techniques in Chapter 3.

Standard conventional hand reflexology treatment

Relax the client's hands by massaging them gently and use a very small amount of non-oily cream. Keep your VRT hand chart available for consultation as you work. It is useful to photocopy the chart and then laminate it to protect it from oils and creams.

Having examined the hands as described on page 11, you are ready to begin the conventional hand reflexology treatment. This should last 15 to 35 minutes. Both you and your client will need to remove watches, bracelets and large rings.

Two options to consider are working first one hand then the other or alternating after every sequence. While practising I suggest that you follow the instructions below and repeat each sequence on the other hand immediately. Once the techniques are familiar you can work one hand thoroughly before moving on to the other.

Greeting the hands

Cup the client's hand, palm upwards, in yours, and massage the hand itself before pulling and gently loosening each finger and thumb one by one. Repeat on the other hand.

Unlike the feet and ankles in particular, the hands are not stiff, and they are not fully supported by the wrists. You must therefore use a firm but gentle grip to work authoritatively and smoothly. The client will also be able to observe all your moves and it is a good idea to practise flowing movements. Remember the rule that your left hand usually supports the client's right hand and your right hand is the working hand and vice versa. Avoid gripping too tightly, but always support the hand firmly.

Working the palm

The client's hand is upright, palm facing you, with their fingers clasped through your fingers (see the illustration on page 15). This enables their hand to be firmly supported but flexible as you inch your thumb across the palm in a criss-cross action so that every reflex is worked. You can flex the hand backwards and forwards, which allows you to stimulate the reflexes firmly but uses less pressure from your own thumb. Frequently change your working hand to access all reflexes. Thirty seconds to a minute is usually enough to stimulate a reflex on the passive hands. You can approach the client's palms with your two hands from behind. Your palms rest on the dorsum of their hand. Curl your fingers and nails to work several reflexes simultaneously.

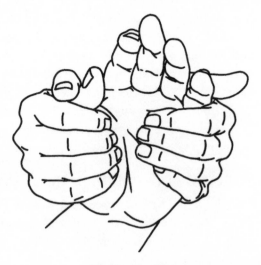

Working the palm

Fingers and thumbs

Use your forefinger and thumb to rotate down the client's fingers and thumb from the base to the nail in tiny moves. Repeat the procedure by pinching the sides of each finger and thumb. Work sensitively, being aware of any granular, hard, puffy or tender parts of the hand. Use cream sparingly. Curl your fingers around the medial (inside) side of the hand and work up the thumb spinal reflexes with your third and fourth fingers. Locate the pituitary reflex (see chart on page 26) with your forefinger and work vigorously.

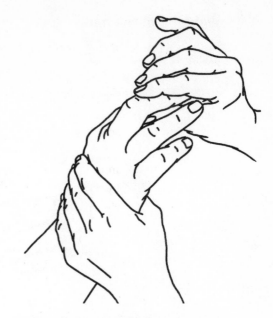

Working the passive fingers and thumbs

Stimulate each nail

Take the client's left hand in your right hand and turn it so it is facing palm down-wards. Place your four fingers underneath their hand, cupping their palm, and put your thumb-tip at wrist level in zone 5 (see page 47) in alignment with the little finger. Pinch down the hand from the wrist in a line along the fifth metacarpal and continue down the finger in small bites until the tip of your thumb-pad touches the fingernail. Arch your thumb, place the tip of your thumbnail at the base of the little fingernail and gently edge the tip of your thumbnail along the centre of their nail to the tip. Repeat, pinching each finger and thumb from the base of the finger to the nail but this time making five passes up the nails so that the tiny zones are generally, not specifically, stimulated. Repeat on other hand.

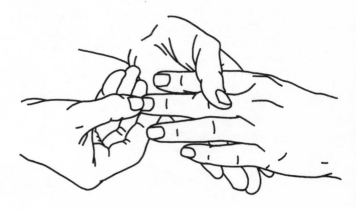

Stimulating each nail

Webbing of the hand

Pinch the webbing between the client's thumb and forefinger and between the
fingers. You will be pinching the palm as you pull your thumb and forefinger
across this loose, fleshy area of the hand. The client can be taught to use this easy
technique as a regular means of self-help to boost the immune system.

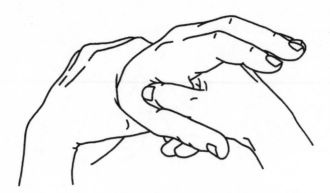

Working the webbing of the hand

Wristband on the hand

Press and work your thumb
across the top of the wrist
several times. You can also
make little caterpillar bites
with your thumb as this will
stimulate the groin,
Fallopian tubes and helper
heart and diaphragm
reflexes as well as the
Zonal Triggers. These are a
deep set of extra reflexes in
the wrists that can dramatically enhance treatment.
For more information see
page 46.

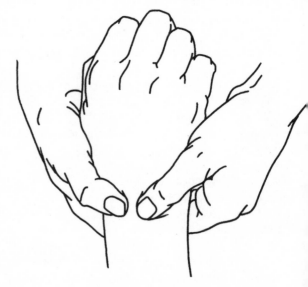

Working the wristband

Kristine Walker and hand reflexology

Kristine Walker is an extremely talented reflexologist and tutor whose teaching, research and clinical practice in this field have been exceptional. Her book *Hand Reflexology* is considered by many to be essential reading for any reflexologist. This chapter has provided ample techniques to work the hands using standard reflexology methods but a fuller picture of the scope of conventional hand reflexology can be obtained from Kristine's book.

Key points to remember

- Hand and foot reflexology are equally powerful but allow a few seconds longer for the hand reflexes to respond.

- Before treatment, wipe both your hands and the client's with a mild antiseptic cloth to freshen and remove any excessive perspiration or stickiness.

- Massage and work the reflexology points on the hands in the resting or passive position for a few minutes before starting VRT.

- Keep a laminated VRT hand chart nearby as you work until you become more familiar with the reflexes.

- Familiarise yourself with further hand reflexology techniques by attending courses or reading comprehensive books on the subject (see Recommended Reading, page 193).

- Ensure your posture is correct and both you and the client are in a comfortable position before the session begins. Be aware if your arms, or the client's, are tiring, and adjust your position.

- The comments on looking after the hands (page 11) apply equally to the therapist and the client.

- Familiarise yourself with any contraindications regarding treatment. If in doubt, do not treat.

- Your knuckles can become as sensitive as your fingertips with practice.

Chapter 3

Basic hand VRT

This chapter gives you the skills to work weight-bearing hands. In only five to ten minutes you can achieve positive results, ranging from release of stress or tension, to aiding the digestive processes or helping to ease a particularly stiff limb or joint. You can use the following step-by-step instructions as your blueprint for all future treatments. This chapter covers all the requirements necessary for offering a comprehensive VRT treatment: first the basic moves, and then beneficial additions for enhancing the basic VRT hand treatment. You will learn:

- Basic hand VRT Sequence
- The Harmonising technique
- Synergistic reflexology
- Diaphragm Rocking
- Zonal Triggers

Once you are more confident you can experiment with the advanced instructions in subsequent chapters. The hands are not as fleshy as the feet and it will take a while to get used to working with a much bonier surface. You will need to develop slightly different techniques for working across the thin, loose skin on the dorsum (top) of the hand. It must be remembered at all times that the hand reflexes are just as sensitive as the feet but the response, once a reflex is triggered, takes a few seconds longer to kick in.

The charts on the following pages contain all the dorsal (top) and plantar (palm) aspects for the hands and feet, and should be referred to throughout the book.

Dorsal hand reflexes

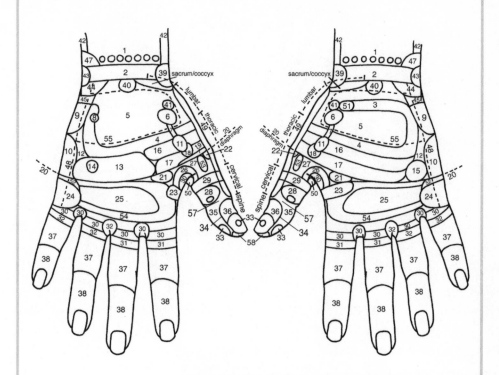

Key master chart for all reflexes

1. Zonal Triggers
2. Fallopian tubes/seminal vesicles/vas deferens/ helper diaphragm/heart
3. Sigmoid
4. Colon
5. Small intestine
6. Bladder
7. Ureter tube
8. Appendix/ileocecal valve
9. Knee
10. Elbow
11. Kidney
12. Helper lateral digestive reflexes
13. Liver
14. Gall bladder
15. Spleen
16. Pancreas
17. Stomach
18. Adrenals
19. Duodenum

20. Diaphragm
21. Solar Plexus
22. Thymus
23. Heart
24. Shoulder
25. Chest/lung/breast
26. Trachea/oesophagus/ bronchial tubes
27. Helper Thyroid
28. Thyroid/parathyroid
29. Neck
30. Lymphatics
31. Eyes
32. Ears/Eustachian tube
33. Pituitary/Pineal/ Hypothalamus
34. Neck - side
35. Brain/skull
36. Face/teeth/ jaws/ tongue/ throat
37. Helper sinuses/teeth
38. Sinuses/brain/skull

39. Uterus/Prostate
40. Helper ovary/testes
41. Penis/vagina
42. Helper lower back/sciatic/ rectum/colon/uterus
43. Ovary/testes
44. Hip/sacro-ileac joint
45. Leg
46. Thoracic area/diaphragm
47. Hip/pelvic area
48. Helper lateral spine
49. Spine
50. Larynx/vocal cords
51. Anus/rectum
52. Armpit
53. Breastbone
54. Ribs
55. Mid/lower back
56. Sciatic nerve
57. Cerebellum/brain stem/ cranial nerves
58. Skull

Palm reflexes

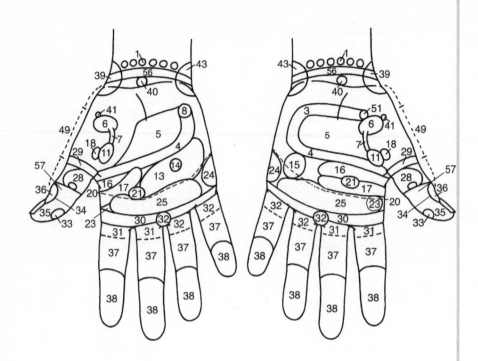

1. Zonal Triggers	23. Heart
	24. Shoulder
3. Sigmoid	25. Chest/lung/breast
4. Colon	26. Trachea/oesophagus/
5. Small intestine	bronchial tubes
6. Bladder	
7. Ureter tube	28. Thyroid/parathyroid
8. Appendix/ileocecal valve	29. Neck
	30. Lymphatics
11. Kidney	31. Eyes
	32. Ears/Eustachian tube
13. Liver	33. Pituitary/pineal/
14. Gall bladder	hypothalamus
15. Spleen	34. Neck – side
16. Pancreas	35. Brain/skull
17. Stomach	36. Face/teeth/ jaws/ tongue/
18. Adrenals	throat
	37. Helper sinuses/teeth
20. Diaphragm	38. Sinuses/brain/skull
21. Solar Plexus	39. Uterus/prostate
	40. Helper ovary/testes
	41. Penis/vagina

43. Ovary/testes

49. Spine

51. Anus/rectum

55. Mid/lower back
56. Sciatic nerve
57. Cerebellum/brain stem/
cranial nerves

Dorsal foot reflexes

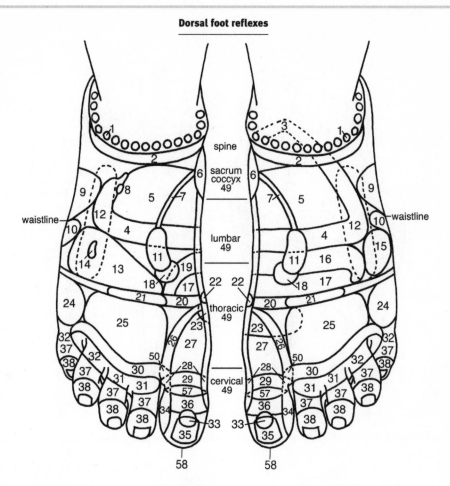

1. Zonal Triggers
2. Fallopian tubes/seminal vesicles/vas deferens/ helper diaphragm/heart
3. Sigmoid
4. Colon
5. Small intestine
6. Bladder
7. Ureter tube
8. Appendix/ileocecal valve
9. Knee
10. Elbow
11. Kidney
12. Helper lateral digestive reflexes
13. Liver
14. Gall bladder
15. Spleen
16. Pancreas
17. Stomach
18. Adrenals
19. Duodenum
20. Diaphragm
21. Solar Plexus
22. Thymus
23. Heart
24. Shoulder
25. Chest/lung/breast
26. Trachea/oesophagus/ bronchial tubes
27. Helper Thyroid
28. Thyroid/parathyroid
29. Neck
30. Lymphatics
31. Eyes
32. Ears/Eustachian tube
33. Pituitary/Pineal/ Hypothalamus
34. Neck – side
35. Brain/skull
36. Face/teeth/ jaws/ tongue/ throat
37. Helper sinuses/teeth
38. Sinuses/brain/skull
49. Spine
50. Larynx/vocal cords

57. Cerebellum/brain stem/ cranial nerves
58. Skull

Plantar foot reflexes

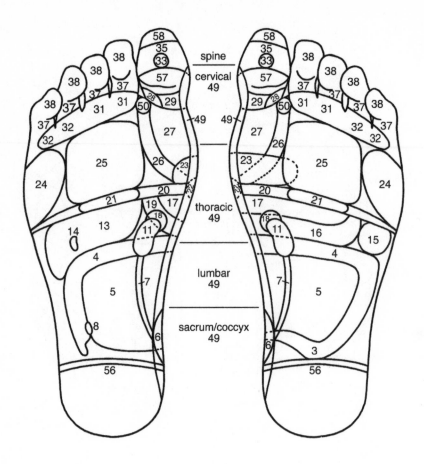

3. Sigmoid
4. Colon
5. Small intestine
6. Bladder
7. Ureter tube
8. Appendix/ileocecal valve

11. Kidney

13. Liver
14. Gall bladder
15. Spleen
16. Pancreas
17. Stomach
18. Adrenals
19. Duodenum

20. Diaphragm
21. Solar plexus
22. Thymus
23. Heart
24. Shoulder
25. Chest/lung/breast
26. Trachea/oesophagus/
    bronchial tubes
27. Helper thyroid
28. Thyroid/parathyroid
29. Neck

31. Eyes
32. Ears/Eustachian tube
33. Pituitary/pineal/
    hypothalamus

35. Brain/skull

37. Helper sinuses/teeth
38. Sinuses/brain/skull

49. Spine
50. Larynx/vocal cords

56. Sciatic nerve
57. Cerebellum/brain
    stem/cranial nerves
58. Skull

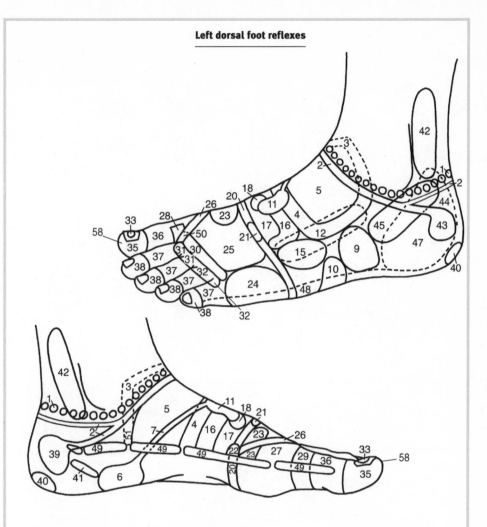

Left dorsal foot reflexes

1. Zonal Triggers
2. Fallopian tubes/ seminal vesicles/vas deferens/helper diaphragm/heart
3. Sigmoid
4. Colon
5. Small intestine
6. Bladder
7. Ureter tube
9. Knee
10. Elbow
11. Kidney
12. Helper lateral digestive reflexes
15. Spleen
16. Pancreas
17. Stomach
18. Adrenals
20. Diaphragm
21. Solar plexus
22. Thymus
23. Heart
24. Shoulder
25. Chest/lung/breast
26. Trachea/oesophagus/ bronchial tubes
27. Helper thyroid
28. Thyroid/parathyroid
29. Neck
30. Lymphatics
31. Eyes
32. Ears/Eustachian tube
33. Pituitary/pineal/ hypothalamus
35. Brain/skull
36. Face/teeth/ jaws/ tongue/ throat
37. Helper sinuses/teeth
38. Sinuses/brain/skull
39. Uterus/prostate
40. Helper ovary/testes
41. Penis/vagina
42. Helper lower back/sciatic/ rectum/colon/uterus
43. Ovary/testes
44. Hip/sacro-iliac joint
45. Leg
47. Hip/pelvic area
48. Helper lateral spine
49. Spine
50. Larynx/vocal cords
58. Skull

Right dorsal reflexes

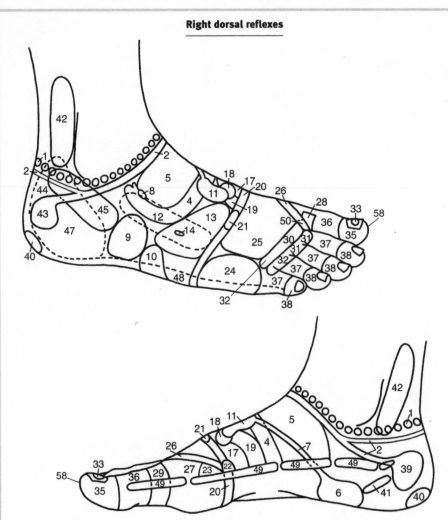

1. Zonal Triggers
2. Fallopian tubes/ seminal vesicles/ vas deferens/helper diaphragm/heart
4. Colon
6. Bladder
7. Ureter tube
8. Appendix/ileocecal valve
9. Knee
10. Elbow
11. Kidney
12. Helper lateral digestive reflexes
13. Liver
14. Gall bladder
17. Stomach
18. Adrenals
19. Duodenum
20. Diaphragm
21. Solar plexus
22. Thymus
23. Heart
24. Shoulder
25. Chest/lung/breast
26. Trachea/oesophagus/ bronchial tubes
27. Helper thyroid
28. Thyroid/parathyroid
29. Neck
30. Lymphatics
31. Eyes
32. Ears/Eustachian tube
33. Pituitary/pineal/ hypothalamus
35. Brain/skull
36. Face/teeth/ jaws/ tongue/ throat
37. Helper sinuses/teeth
38. Sinuses/brain/skull
39. Uterus/prostate
40. Helper ovary/testes
41. Penis/vagina
42. Helper lower back/sciatic/ rectum/colon/uterus
43. Ovary/testes
44. Hip/sacro-iliac joint
45. Leg
47. Hip/pelvic area
48. Helper lateral spine
49. Spine
50. Larynx/vocal cords

58. Skull

Thoracic calf reflexes on the leg

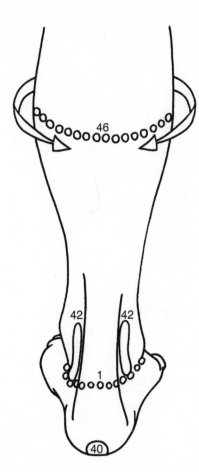

1. Zonal Triggers

40. Helper ovary/testes

42. Helper lower back/sciatic/
    rectum/colon/uterus

46. Thoracic area/diaphragm

Thoracic calf reflexes on the arm

1. Zonal Triggers
39. Uterus/prostate
40. Helper ovary/testes
42. Helper lower back/sciatic/
    rectum/colon/uterus
43. Ovary/testes
46. Thoracic area/diaphragm

The key rule with VRT is to back off once a painful reflex has been contacted and then gently stimulate the area in a rotating movement for a maximum of 30 seconds per reflex. Hand VRT is very quick and effective in its own right but ideally it should be used for a few minutes either side of a conventional hand reflexology session.

The shortened but comprehensive hand treatment is invaluable for treating the elderly, chronically ill and children, who are not always suited to a longer session. If you offer reflexology in the workplace, in a hospice or similar, the quick treatments allow you to double the number of people you can treat in a given time without compromising on results. VRT is a very powerful and flexible form of reflexology that should normally not take more than about eight to ten minutes in total if used as part of traditional hand reflexology.

VRT variation of treatments

The basic five-minute treatment can be used:

- In its own right.
- Before and after treating a client in the conventional hand reflexology manner.
- As part of a shortened 20-minute complete VRT treatment.
- As first aid, in which case only the spinal and pelvic reflexes are worked, followed by specific advanced techniques.
- When specific priority reflexes are worked for self-help on the hands, feet and nails.

The following basic VRT hand treatment is a short sequence and each session should take a maximum of four to five minutes. It may take you longer in the early practice stages, but while learning be careful not to overwork any particular reflex.

The key to VRT, in general, is always to begin by working the spine/central nervous system reflexes, which are situated on the medial (inside) edges of the hands or feet. You will also need to work around the wrists or ankles to activate the powerful Zonal Triggers described in this chapter.

> **A key point to remember**
>
> It is important not to overwork a limb if it happens to gain more mobility during a VRT treatment. VRT tutors always counsel caution at first when a limb has freed up, as the muscles and ligaments need time to fully heal.

Preparation for basic hand VRT

- Take a case history and ascertain if there are any problems that may affect the use of VRT, such as giddiness or problems connected with standing for any length of time. Ensure that the weight-bearing hands or arms will not experience discomfort when leaned on. Check first with the person you are treating to ensure that they have no conditions of which you were not aware.
- If dealing with an orthopaedic condition, the range of mobility should be tested before and after the session.
- Prepare yourself and the seating areas as described on page 34.
- Remember that it is essential when working on a client that both hands are treated alternately at every stage. VRT is extremely powerful and the body needs to be kept in balance by repeatedly stimulating the reflexes on either side of the body. The only VRT exception is when you are using the self-help techniques, as the body is working within your own energy field and can cope with the stimulation of a complete hand at a time.

The correct VRT hand position

Always ensure that the person treated is initially seated on an upright chair with their arms leaning on a cushion on the table. Alternatively, they can sit facing you and you can place their hands on a cushion on your lap. On some occasions they will be standing with their hand pressed on a table for a short VRT hand first-aid treatment. Hand VRT is particularly useful if the reflexologist has a physical impediment and cannot kneel. In this case when weight-bearing hand and foot VRT are used in the same session, the client can stand and put one foot at a time on a chair. The therapist can sit on an adjacent chair, or use a small stool, to work in this manner. Another option is for the client to sit and place their hands forwards on a low table, while you kneel on a cushion in front of them. Instead of kneeling, you can also use a sloping stool that stands about 15 cm off the ground.

Client being treated in a standing position

The correct posture for the practitioner

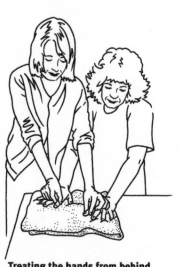

Treating the hands from behind

Be prepared to work the client's hands from behind if necessary to gain the best results. This involves standing behind the standing client; or you can sit alongside them when seated and place both of your hands on either side of the client's hand with your thumbs on the dorsum (top) of the hand and your fingers ready to work the upright palm. A cushion must always be available for the therapist to kneel on for working the hands and feet at the same time. Bad posture caused by twisting to reach the hand instead of moving gently can cause unnecessary pressure on the back, wrists, hands and shoulders. A client can be asked to move slightly when their weight-bearing arm is in the correct position.

The golden rule for VRT

Never ask anyone to stand on a stool, chair, stairs or box if you are going to treat their hands and feet at the same time (this is called synergistic reflexology, or synergistic VRT). VRT is very powerful and there is a rare possibility that someone could become light-headed or dizzy and fall if they were in a slightly elevated position. If you are incapacitated and cannot kneel, then opt to treat their foot resting on a chair seat beside you or:

● Treat the weight-bearing hands only.

● Accept that hand and foot VRT is not for you.

● Pass your client onto another trained VRT reflexologist.

Basic method for VRT on the hands

It does not matter with which hand you start but for continuity here I will usually start with the right. First, arrange the client's elbows on the cushion for comfort as you massage and relax the hands before commencing the VRT treatment. This has the effect of stimulating the deep zonal wrist reflexes, which makes the entire body more responsive to VRT. The client then firmly presses their palm on a flat surface with the arm straight.

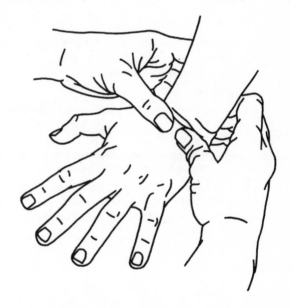

Working the wrists on the weight-bearing hand

Wrist reflexes including Zonal Triggers

Key steps

● Always start with the wrist reflexes. Sit or stand and face the client's hands.

● Work under and over the wrist bones simultaneously on both the dorsal (upper) and palm side of the hand.

● Always slide your thumb and caterpillar walk it backwards and forwards across the wrist bracelet to activate the Zonal Triggers and helper heart/diaphragm reflexes.

● Stimulate the pelvic and hip reflexes.

● Work your fingers simultaneously up either side of the wrists to at least 8 cm up the arm – this stimulates the sciatic reflexes. Repeat on the left hand.

● The next three moves – the Lumbar Spine Release and working/tapping the spinal reflexes – should be applied consecutively to the right hand and then the left hand.

Medial (inside) edge of the hand – Lumbar Spine Release

This action of pulling the spinal reflexes a fraction stimulates the vertebrae, muscular and neural pathway reflexes, and can ease lower back pain.

Key steps

● Move sideways to the client. Support the top of their hand with your left palm and with your right fingertips firmly press the medial (inside) side of their thumb. Your thumb steadies the client's thumb. Pull gently upwards a millimetre or two with your right hand and release. Repeat three times on both hands.

● Do not move your fingers under the metacarpal thumb bone – they are just acting as a gentle lever. Pull gently upwards as if to make a 'banana' shape. Do not move or work your fingers that are hooked under the client's hand.

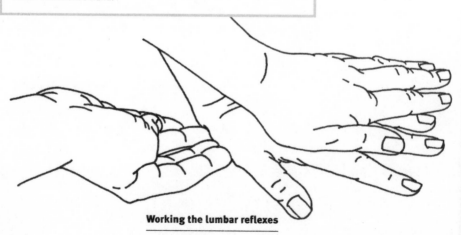

Working the lumbar reflexes

Medial (inside) edge hand – work the spinal reflexes

These moves can ease back pain and stimulate the nervous system.

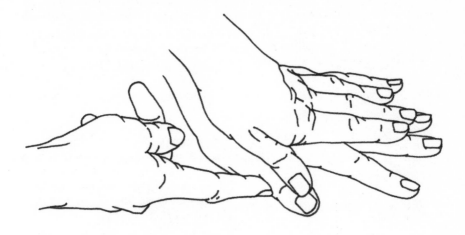

Working the spinal reflexes

Key steps
- Caterpillar walk with your index finger or use four fingers to work down the length of the spinal reflexes, pressing each reflex until your little finger reaches the cervical reflexes.
- Repeat three times.
- Tap up and down the spinal reflexes with four fingers three times.
- Ask your client to then turn sideways facing the other way so that they can place their other hand at the correct angle for working the three spinal moves above.

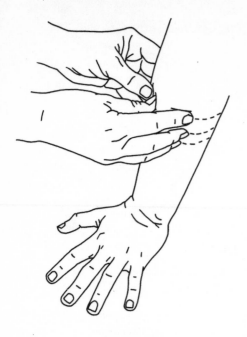

Thoracic release

Reflexes on the lower arm (radius/ulna bones) – thoracic release

Working the series of reflex points around the widest section of the lower arm (the radius and ulna bones) can help to relax the thoracic spine area, and is helpful for asthmatics.

Key steps
- Locate the widest circumference of the lower arm and work the lower arm reflexes from back to front, using a fairly casual pinching and pressing movement with your fingers and thumbs of both hands.

- Work this area once or twice then repeat on the other arm.

Working the fingers and thumbs – head and neck area

With this technique, the brain, sinuses, ears, eyes, neck and thyroid gland are all triggered when the fingers and thumbs are worked. Tiny subtle reflexes connected with the teeth, larynx and throat are also worked. Remind your client to ensure their hands are weight-bearing.

Repeat the sequence once or twice for chronic sinus and other head conditions.

Key steps
- Stand or sit in front of the hands. Working both hands at once, simultaneously pinch up and down the sides of each thumb, then rotate your two index fingers in a firm, circular movement over the tops of both thumbs from the nail to the base of the thumbs and then repeat these moves on each finger in turn.

- Keep the fingers splayed open as far as possible without straining them.

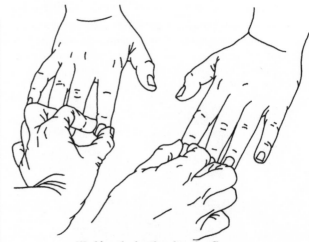

Working the head and neck reflexes

Working the bases of the fingers and thumbs – lymphatic, chest and lung rotation

This technique stimulates the immune system, and works best with a little cream. Working the chest/lung reflexes is helpful in cases of asthma or respiratory conditions.

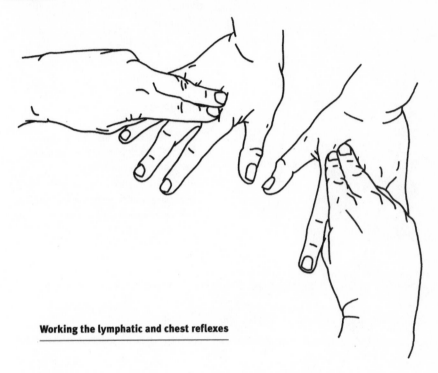

Working the lymphatic and chest reflexes

Key steps

- Work both hands simultaneously. Place your index and third fingers at the bases of the client's thumbs and, in a circular movement, simultaneously work the lymphatic reflexes at the base of each finger where they join the metacarpal area of the hand. Spread the rotation outwards to cover the chest/lung reflexes as well.

- Either return to the bases of the thumbs and repeat the operation or work the same movements in reverse starting at the bases of the little fingers.

Mid-base of the wrist – ovary and testes helper reflex

To work the ovary/testes reflex, ask the client to point their weight-bearing hands away from you, giving you access to the bases of their palms at the heel of the hand. The ovary/testes point is also an energiser and can be used in a totally different context on children to help to control allergic reactions.

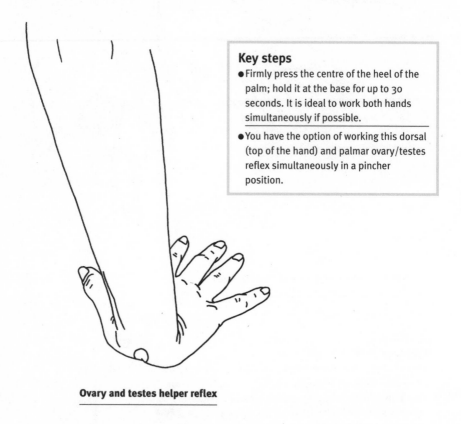

Key steps

- Firmly press the centre of the heel of the palm; hold it at the base for up to 30 seconds. It is ideal to work both hands simultaneously if possible.
- You have the option of working this dorsal (top of the hand) and palmar ovary/testes reflex simultaneously in a pincher position.

Ovary and testes helper reflex

Return to the wrist reflexes

Return at least once during the VRT treatment to work the Zonal Trigger and other reflexes on the wrists briefly to stimulate the body.

Finger walk the top of the hand (metacarpals)

The hands can be approached from the side or behind for this movement. This theory works on the premise that VRT triggers all the Fitzgerald zones (see page 3) into action, thus energising the same reflexes on the palm and dorsal (upper) sides of the hands.

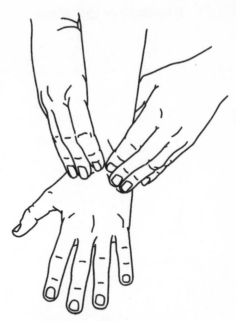

Key steps
- Point your index fingers so that they touch with your hands forming a V-shape.
- Move the fingers swiftly down the metacarpals from the wrist to the fingertips.
- Make sure every part of the top of the hand is stimulated by making at least three passes – this action is also treating every organ and gland in the body.
- Glide off the fingertips.

Finger walking the metacarpals

Pituitary Pinch

This is an extremely powerful reflex point that is useful in helping to stabilise hormonal imbalances in men and women. It can also have a relaxing effect, often producing an instant feeling of warmth throughout the body.

Key steps
- Place your forefingers under the client's thumbs with your nails touching the flat surfaces. The client's thumb-pads will be naturally splayed on their sides at a slight angle to the table.
- Place your thumb-pads on the client's thumbnails with your thumbs and press firmly.
- Ensure the client is applying extra pressure to their thumbs for 30 seconds as they gently push downwards a fraction.
- Work both reflexes simultaneously where possible.

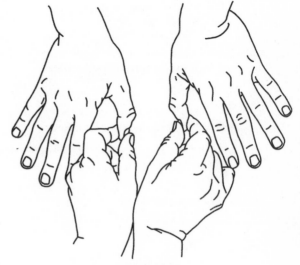

Pituitary pinch

Harmoniser technique

This is a very useful and effective balancing technique and should be used at the end of every treatment. It can also be applied during a session (weight-bearing or conventional) if a client reports a strong reaction.

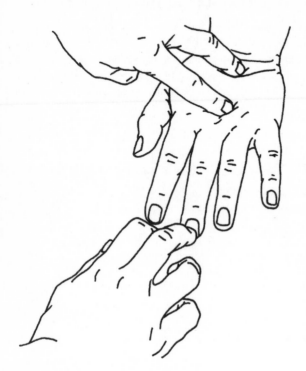

With the third fingernail of one hand, press the middle point of the client's nail on the middle finger. Use the index and third finger of your other hand for the following moves:

1. Press the dorsal solar plexus reflex with your thumb or finger-tip and hold.

2. Press the Zonal Trigger in zone 3 (see page 47) with your finger-tip, and simultaneously hold all three reflexes for 15 to 30 seconds. This point is found by simply aligning the two reflexes.

3. Repeat on the other hand immediately. Repeat twice if necessary. This can help to consolidate your work and will also immediately calm the body and prevent any over-reaction.

The Harmoniser

When I developed the Harmoniser technique I did not specify that the therapist's right nail should touch the client's right nail. My feeling was that either hand would suffice. Feedback from tutors and my own research suggests that the Harmoniser effect may be enhanced when the nail is worked by either your corresponding right nail or your left nail.

See Chapter 6 for self-help instructions.

THE HARMONISER HELPS EAR, NOSE AND THROAT PATIENTS

A reflexologist in Sussex often has ear, nose and throat patients referred to her by a doctor specialising in those conditions. She found VRT could be too powerful for some clients, as they sometimes felt unbalanced when the delicate ear reflexes were worked. She reports that, since using the Harmoniser, she can now confidently give these clients VRT, as they no longer overreact to a treatment.

While I was teaching a course in the Netherlands a reflexologist was given a VRT treatment by a colleague. The treatment had freed up her stiff shoulder, and as she was showing off her new-found mobility to the group, she began to feel faint. I applied the Harmoniser to her partially weight-bearing feet as she sat. Immediately I felt a pulse in the reflexes and she took a deep breath as colour rushed back to her cheeks. Within five minutes she was feeling well and went back into the practical lesson. This technique is equally effective on the hands and very accessible in times of emergency.

Powerful techniques to enhance the basic VRT hand treatment

The treatment you have learnt in the first part of this chapter is the model for all VRT hand sessions. The second part shows you how to enhance your treatments by introducing more powerful techniques to consolidate your work. Always remember the following points:

- For chronic (long-standing) conditions work the reflexes no more than two to three times weekly as the body needs time to regenerate.
- Acute conditions can be worked daily if the schedule permits.
- Self-help VRT can be administered several times a day. The client can be taught self-help VRT techniques on the feet or hands to stimulate the immune system, or help a particular condition, in between treatments.

The VRT advanced technique options

1. My preferred option is to always treat the hands at the beginning and end of a session. The basic VRT techniques make the entire body more receptive to conventional hand reflexology. The advanced techniques are applied at the end to consolidate the treatment.
2. Use VRT at the beginning or end of a session but not both. Some therapists give VRT at the commencement of a session to prime the body before conventional reflexology. Others wait until they have more information

from the client about their responses, and then apply specific advanced techniques towards the end of the session.

3. VRT first aid involves briefly working the wrists and spinal reflexes only, immediately followed by synergistic work on two or three reflexes (see below) and optional advanced techniques.

Synergistic reflexology

Synergistic means the increased effect of two factors working together in cooperation. Synergistic reflexology utilises and concentrates the energetic impulse from the corresponding reflexes in the hands and feet and accelerates the healing process. When a reflex on the hand is simultaneously worked with the identical reflex on the foot it accelerates the effects of VRT – as it is a means of *turning up the power* in the body. During the treatment you will have ascertained what priority conditions need treating synergistically and you will be targeting this energy to the parts of the body most in need. Synergistic reflexology is easy to apply as you simply find the same points on the feet and the hands and work the two together for a maximum of 30 seconds. The client must ideally be in a standing position for synergistic reflexology, and you should kneel on a cushion to work the weight-bearing feet.

Synergistic reflexology is powerful and should be used sparingly at the end of a treatment to work up to three priority reflexes only. Any more would cause the body to dissipate its energies in too many directions at once, possibly causing a mild headache or nausea. Synergistic reflexology takes the separate benefits of hand and foot reflexology three stages further by:

- **Simultaneously working the same reflexes on the hand and foot when the client is standing.** This is the standard mode of applying synergistic reflexology at the end of a treatment, whether it is a five-minute basic VRT, the 15- to 25-minute complete hand VRT or a combined VRT/conventional reflexology session.

- **Using the reclining position.** This is much more subtle as weight-bearing is not involved and several reflexes can be prioritised this way during a conventional treatment.

- **Simultaneously working the weight-bearing hands (palm downwards) and the standing feet.** This is only used occasionally for intransigent problems that have not responded to the other methods. See the illustration on page 34 for details.

Method

The hands are worked first for a few minutes' basic VRT, at the beginning of the shortened complete or full hand reflexology treatment.

Three reflexes will have been selected as priority areas for extra help. The top priority reflex will be worked last with a third reflex, the Zonal Trigger, as well, on both hands and feet.

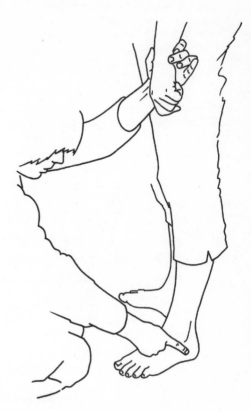

1. Select one of the reflexes to be worked synergistically, for example the ovary/testes reflex. Work it on the passive hand as a first choice, or on the weight-bearing dorsum (top) of the hand if you are treating an intractable problem. It is not easy to work the hands and feet at the same time when the hand is weight-bearing, as you have to stretch at a slightly odd angle to find the reflex point.

2. Find the hand reflex corresponding to the foot reflex. Start with the priority reflex if a one-sided problem. Rotate your finger on the reflexes for a few seconds and hold for 30 seconds maximum.

Working two reflexes synergistically

3. Repeat this procedure on the other hand and foot. In the case of the liver, for example, there is no corresponding reflex on the left hand or foot but you would always work the identical shadow reflex area to ensure that the zones are balanced.

4. Select a second priority hand reflex and repeat the procedure.

5. Select the top priority reflex and work the hand and foot reflexes together for a few seconds before locating the third reflex, the Zonal Trigger (see page 46).

Be aware of the different proportions of
the hands and feet in relation to the body
reflexes. For example, the cervical reflexes
on the thumb are much further apart than
on the smaller big toe.

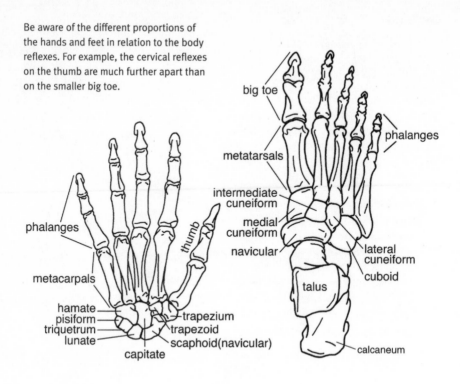

The bones of the hands and feet

Zonal Triggers

Zonal Triggers are a deep set of extra reflexes forming a circle around the wrists
and ankles that have enabled reflexologists to fine-tune and enhance their treatments. This series of tiny reflexes can only be accessed when worked in
conjunction with other specific reflexes on the hands and feet. It seems that by
working these Zonal Trigger reflexes, in conjunction with a priority reflex on the
hand or foot, not only does a particular part of the body respond, but all organs,
glands or skeletal reflexes in that zone react positively to this brief stimulation.

The zone theory states that the body is divided into ten longitudinal zones,
which are mirrored on the hands and feet, with five on each hand and foot. There
are also four transverse zones across the hands and feet, which mark the shoulder
girdle, diaphragm, waistline and pelvic floor (see the illustration on page 2). The
flows of energy throughout the body are directed through these ten zones. VRT
appears to decongest the zones very quickly by accessing the body's own healing
mechanisms, thus allowing energy to flow through unimpeded to the target area.

The VRT wrist and ankle reflexes are extremely important as a 'window' into the body. I suggest that there are three layers of specific reflexes around the wrists and ankles that can be accessed according to bodily needs. Zonal Triggers are the third and deepest layer of reflexes. By working this band precisely, the Zonal Trigger reflex is usually found to be more sensitive than the others and it is often, but not always, in the same zone as the main organ, gland or joint being treated.

The Zonal Trigger reflexes and other reflexes should be visualised as follows:

1. **Top layer of wrist reflexes** Conventional lymph and groin/Fallopian tubes/vas deferens/seminal vesicle.

2. **Middle layer of wrist reflexes** VRT helper diaphragm (left and right hand) and helper heart (left hand). These heart reflexes are useful to work in a secondary capacity.

3. **Deepest layer of wrist reflexes** These Zonal Trigger reflexes are activated when worked simultaneously with another reflex that relates to a specific part of the body.

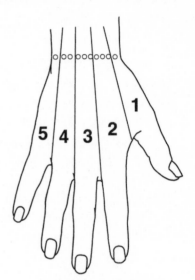

Zonal Triggers and zones

The cross-section of the hand shows:

1. The nail reflexes

2. The dorsal reflexes

3. The emotional layer of reflexes

4. The body's catalogue of past injuries, illness and ageing

5. Palm reflexes

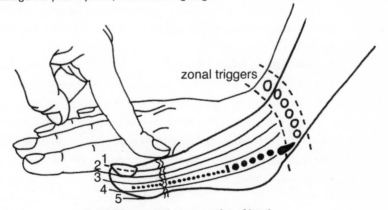

Zonal Triggers and cross-section of hand

Balancing the body and 30-second VRT rule

- This is one of the key rules for all aspects of VRT: never work a weight-bearing reflex for over 30 seconds at any time. Any longer is unnecessary and can cause over-stimulation.

- Always work the corresponding reflexes on both hands to balance the body. If the reflex is only on one hand or foot, such as the heart on the left hand or the liver on the right, then work the identical corresponding shadow area to balance the body via the zones.

Prioritising a reflex using Zonal Triggers

Working the Zonal Triggers is an extension of synergistic reflexology where the same hand and foot reflexes are worked simultaneously. First locate the appropriate hand and foot reflex, then the Zonal Trigger, which is located around the wrist or ankle-band; these two points are then worked on the foot while a third is worked on the hand. The hand can also be used to work two reflexes simultaneously. These triggers work by increasing the power, or stimulation, from the reflexes to the part of the body in most need of attention.

This is a very powerful technique that should only be used once during a treatment as it channels extra energy to a priority area of the body.

The only time Zonal Triggers can be used more than once in a treatment is if you access two reflexes in the same system such as the pituitary and the adrenal glands (endocrine system) or the stomach and the bowel (digestive system).

Do not be tempted to work extra three-point techniques on other systems of the body when the client is standing, as it could produce a mild healing crisis if the body attempted to channel extra energy in too many directions at once. The energising effects of Zonal Triggers are much more subtle when the client is in the reclining position. As the result is not so powerful the Zonal Triggers can be connected to several systems.

Ideally the Zonal Trigger will be worked at the end of a treatment. This could be directly after the basic VRT, the shorter complete VRT, or a VRT/conventional treatment of varying duration. The recommended application of Zonal Trigger techniques follows the following format.

Zonal Trigger treatment format

- Basic VRT for three to five minutes at the beginning of a 35-minute conventional hand reflexology treatment.

- Follow this with a brief return to VRT techniques (up to five minutes) at the end of the session. Select two synergistic reflexes as secondary areas for help and one Zonal Trigger, which will be the key priority reflex.

- At the completion of a VRT treatment you may wish to add several of the advanced techniques found in this chapter.

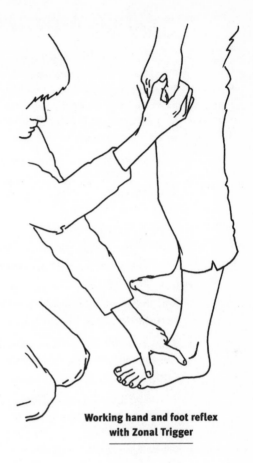

Working hand and foot reflex with Zonal Trigger

Finding a Zonal Trigger

You can start with either hand but for continuity the right hand and foot will be used for this example.

Method 1: hand VRT using the passive hand for the priority reflex and connecting it with the corresponding reflex and Zonal Trigger situated on the foot.

Decide which priority reflex to work. Two other priority reflexes will be worked synergistically but without the Zonal Trigger. For illustration the shoulder reflex will be worked on.

1. Work the hand and foot shoulder reflexes simultaneously for a few seconds. If you are treating a one-sided problem always start work on the hand that connects with the weak part of the body.

2. Temporarily let go of the hand reflex and continue to hold the shoulder reflex on the foot. With your other free hand carefully work your index finger around the ankle-band in tiny bites starting at the back of the foot around the ankle. At some point, usually in the same zone as the reflex you are pressing, the client will feel a

tiny pinprick. This very distinct pressure indicates that you have found the Zonal Trigger.

3. If you fail to find a Zonal Trigger in the corresponding zone, keep working around the ankle until you locate a pinprick spot and hold it. If you cannot find a Zonal Trigger point on the ankle-band, return to the correct zone, in line with the priority index, and hold that point with your index finger. If you find more than one pinprick reflex in the same zone, work each one for a few seconds to ascertain which is the most tender, then work the identified key reflex on the foot.

4. Press the Zonal Trigger reflex on the ankle with your index finger and use it like a pivot as your thumb (same hand) touches the shoulder reflex on the foot. Stimulate the two reflexes together for a few seconds and hold for a maximum of 30 seconds.

5. Reach up from your kneeling position and relocate the shoulder reflex on the dorsum (top) of the passive hand below the little finger, stimulate briefly, and hold the three points together for 30 seconds.

6. If you are working on an intransigent problem that needs more powerful help, work the weight-bearing hand and weight-bearing foot. For most conditions you will work the passive hand and weight-bearing foot.

7. If you were treating someone who was bedridden, you could work the reclining foot and then ask them to weight-bear their hand on a small bedside table. It is even possible to ask them to press firmly on their leg or a mattress.

8. Repeat on the left hand and foot in the same manner. Always work the same reflexes on both hands and feet to balance the zonal energy. Never work two different Zonal Triggers on the right and left hand because it will put the body out of balance.

9. If the client is in a reclining position it is perfectly acceptable to work several Zonal Trigger combinations of three reflexes during one treatment, as long as both hands and feet are worked each time because the energy is subtle and not as powerful as when standing.

Method 2: hand VRT using the priority reflex and Zonal Trigger on the weight-bearing hand and the corresponding reflex on the weight-bearing foot.

1. Select the reflex on the weight-bearing hand, for example the shoulder, and allow the client's hand to remain weight-bearing on a table. Now access their hand Zonal Trigger connected with the shoulder reflex by finding a pinprick sensation around the wrist area – usually in zone 5 (see page 47) in this case.

2. Kneel down and work the shoulder reflex in zone 5 on the weight-bearing foot. Stimulate all three reflexes simultaneously for a few seconds and hold for a maximum of 30 seconds.

3. Repeat on the other hand and foot.

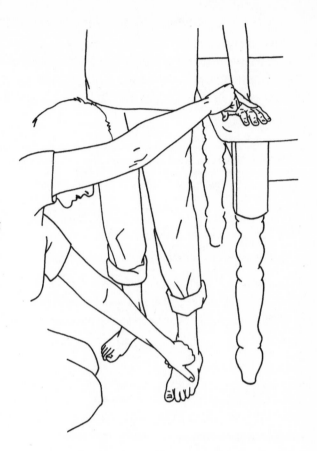

Working the weight-bearing hands and feet

Posture

Synergistic reflexology is easy to apply, as the client's arms will be naturally hanging downwards beside their body. VRT is a short treatment so it is possible for you to sit or kneel comfortably on the floor as you simultaneously press a foot and hand reflex. If you cannot kneel yourself for any reason and your client is agile enough to raise their foot to rest on a chair seat, you can treat their weight-bearing foot by sitting on another chair beside them and working their feet one by one. They should lean forwards and put weight on the foot that is being worked. Do not attempt this if a client is immobile, elderly or prone to dizziness.

Guidelines for working referral reflexes

By working the appropriate reflexes on the hands or feet you can consolidate your work by stimulating the reflexes on the actual parts of the body. For example, if someone twists their right ankle, do not touch the painful ankle itself but vigorously work the corresponding reflexes on their right wrist. Remember the rule on zones:

- The wrist corresponds to the ankle.

- The individual fingers correspond to the individual toes.

- The palm corresponds to the sole.

- The heel of the palm corresponds to the heel of the foot.

- The spinal hand reflexes run from the outer side of the thumb to the wrist.

- The spinal foot reflexes run from the outer edge of the big toe to the heel.

- The discrepancy between the length of the big toe and the thumb means that the hand cervical reflexes are wider apart than those on the feet and the thoracic and lumbar reflexes are much closer together.

Diaphragm Rocking

Diaphragm Rocking is a a very effective technique that is deeply relaxing and appears to pump energy to the part of the body that is most in need of help at any particular moment. The effectiveness of VRT is enhanced when Diaphragm Rocking techniques are applied to the passive hand. Diaphragm Rocking can deeply relax and balance the body very quickly and at the same time appears to target the organ or area most in need of healing within the body. It also energises the therapist.

I devised this technique originally to combat insomnia, as it was very effective in resetting the body clock. The rocking movement has been very helpful in cases of trauma, deep stress, addiction and chronic illness which will not respond to conventional complementary treatments. When applying Diaphragm Rocking, I often become aware of warmth in my chest or sternum area and I feel calm and relaxed. I have concluded that this gentle rocking, over a period of one to four minutes, sets up an exchange of neutral energy between the therapist and the person being worked on.

Diaphragm Rocking can be used in every reflexology treatment whether VRT is introduced or not. In my opinion the effect of Diaphragm Rocking is as profound as the effect of VRT. Both accelerate the healing properties that lie within the body. Zonal Triggers, synergistic reflexology and other techniques enhance the VRT, however Diaphragm Rocking can override the key reflexes a reflexologist has chosen to work, as shown in the example below.

A partner or parent can easily learn to work the hands or feet of someone preparing to go to sleep – others, including children, can be taught to treat their own hands by very effective self-help Diaphragm Rocking movements (see Chapter 6).

Diaphragm Rocking can be used in the following modes

- Applied and self-help on the hands to induce sleep.

- After a five-minute basic VRT treatment to consolidate the session.

- Halfway through the shortened complete hand VRT treatment that lasts approximately 15 to 20 minutes.

- Included in the full conventional hand reflexology treatment, which comprises a 30- to 35-minute session.

- In any VRT foot reflexology treatment in all the permutations that apply to the hands.

Method for Diaphragm hand rocking

The client sits opposite you, ideally across a small table, with their right arm resting on a cushion and their palm facing downwards. Diaphragm Rocking can also be administered in the standing position.

1. Using both your hands, lift the client's hand so their palm is facing you and the fingers are pointing upwards. Bend and flip the hand backwards and forwards from the wrist to achieve the full range of mobility.

2. Place both your flat thumbs horizontally to the wrist slightly medial to the mid-point on the diaphragm line and meeting on the solar plexus reflex.

3. Place the four fingers of your hands on the top of the client's hand so that they touch, making a V-shape pointing towards their body.

4. While fully supporting their hand push your flat thumbs into the flesh of their palm and rock their hand backwards and forwards.

5. Press the dorsum (top of the hand) firmly and slide your fingers outwards a fraction to 'fan' and stretch the metacarpals as the client's hand is pulled towards you. The key technique here is to gently press your index fingers into the hand, making it slightly concave, and produce a distinctive rolling, relaxing sensation. As your fingers press on the top (dorsum) of the hand ensure that your thumbs release so that the person only experiences pressure on one side of the hand at any one time.

6. Pull the client's hand towards you, take the pressure off the metacarpals, press the solar plexus reflex with your two horizontal thumbs, and push the hand back towards their body. Never squeeze the hand.

7. Once a rhythm is obtained, rock the hand gently for at least 15 rocks per hand. This should be visualised as a pumping action, with energy being pumped around the body to the area of greatest need. Make 15 rocking actions on each hand but you can continue for up to two minutes per hand in cases of deep trauma or stress.

8. Ensure you sit upright in your chair as you work and allow your elbows to bend outwards and upwards as you rock the feet.

9. Diaphragm Rocking is deeply relaxing but it is important that the person does not unwind too quickly as the therapist needs some feedback while the reflexes are worked. The best solution is to introduce the Diaphragm Rocking roughly halfway through the treatment. The client often relaxes so quickly and deeply that they cannot help but fall asleep or doze.

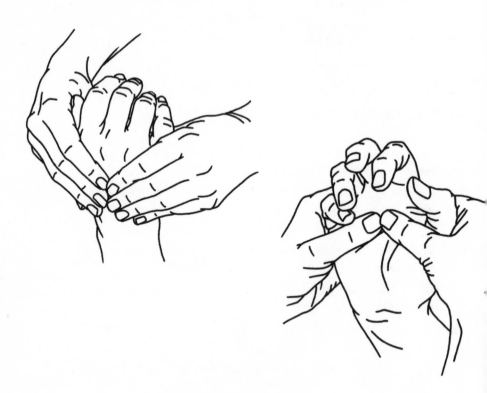

Diaphragm Rocking technique

Diaphragm Rocking can guide a therapist to the root cause of a problem

A client came to me with a sore, stiff shoulder, for which he had been given a steroid injection by his GP to ease the pain. As I used Diaphragm Rocking during his reflexology/VRT treatment he reported that his neck had become warm, not the shoulder, as I would have anticipated given the medical diagnosis.
Subsequent X-rays showed that it was a cervical vertebra problem in his neck that was causing the pain in the shoulder. The Diaphragm Rocking seemed to trigger the body's own innate healing properties to target the correct part of his skeletal system.

PRACTITIONER'S CASE STUDY

Condition: Panic attack/asthma.
Client: Male. **Aged:** 55.
Duration of illness: 5 minutes.
Aim of treatment: To redress a critical situation – an injured deep-sea diver was experiencing severe breathing difficulties.
Result: Impressive. He recovered after approximately two minutes of Diaphragm Rocking.
Practitioner's comments: While diving several kilometres out to sea, a slightly overweight gentleman was pulled aboard with a cut leg, having suffered an asthmatic panic attack. He lay on the deck gasping for air and deteriorating rapidly. With no medical aid available I set to work on his feet with the Diaphragm Rocking technique to calm the system and to prioritise energy to where it was needed most. Within two minutes the man was sitting up, fully recovered and breathing normally.
Author's comment: This is an exceptional report of the power of Diaphragm Rocking, a very simple technique that complements VRT. Previously, when this man had experienced these attacks, he was hospitalised for emergency resuscitation but Diaphragm Rocking enabled his own body to quickly regain control.

Guidelines for full VRT treatment

VRT is a profound and effective treatment. Do not treat for more than five minutes maximum in any one session, without the break of a passive treatment in between. Maximum time would normally be three to five minutes of VRT at the beginning of the session, and the same at the end, to finish a treatment. Hand VRT can be combined with conventional foot reflexology.

Apply the basic VRT treatment step by step – remember to keep alternating the hands. (See page 35.)

1. **Synergistic reflexology.** Select a maximum of three priority reflexes and work the identical reflexes on the hand and foot at the same time. Always work both the left and the right hands to balance the body, even if it is a right- or left-sided problem only.

2. One of the three reflexes selected will be the priority reflex: work one Zonal Trigger and the synergistic reflexology reflexes for the priority condition. Add selected advanced and nail-working techniques from Chapters 4 and 5.

3. Pituitary Pinch – hold for 30 seconds.

4. To conclude: apply the Harmoniser technique. If the client is sensitive or has felt a reaction, repeat this procedure two or three times to centre and relax the body.

Key points to remember

- Surroundings: use a table or other hard surface to lean on, and a quiet workroom with no telephone to cause a distraction.

- Equipment: use a towel or mat on which the client stands for synergistic reflexology, antiseptic wipes and non-oily cream (optional). You will also need a cushion to kneel on for the Diaphragm Rocking technique. Make sure your hands are smooth and clean, with short fingernails.

- Check there are no physical contraindicated conditions such a rash or problem with the arm, hands or wrist itself. For general contraindications see the guidelines in Chapter 1, page 8.

- Aim for good posture as you work. If possible, let the client turn so you can work the hands in different positions.

- Always start with the wrist/spinal reflexes and keep alternating the hands.

- Remember to firmly support the client's hand with your other hand whenever possible.

- Return to the wrist reflexes at least once during a treatment to refresh and stimulate the Zonal Triggers.

- VRT can be a very pleasurable and gentle experience but it can also be temporarily quite painful. Tune into your client's needs and be ready to back off and work more gently if necessary.

- As you work make a mental note of the two reflexes you will work synergistically and the priority reflex that you will work with synergistic reflexology and the Zonal Triggers.

- Always conclude with the balancing and very effective Harmoniser technique and remember it can be freely applied within all treatments whether reclining or weight-bearing.

- Always warn a client that they may feel energised but equally they may feel tired or possibly experience a mild headache after a treatment.

- Advise everyone to drink more water generally, but especially after a treatment to flush out any impurities and to help prevent headaches.

- Use the Zonal Triggers during every treatment, whether conventional or VRT, to greatly enhance your results.

- Do not work a reflex for longer than 30 seconds. The reflexes should be stimulated for a few seconds, then held with slight pressure.

Chapter 4

Advanced VRT hand techniques

This chapter teaches advanced techniques for the hands that will enhance the basic VRT treatment. There are some conditions that do not respond as quickly as anticipated to a normal treatment; the techniques you will learn in this chapter can help to accelerate the healing processes. It is advisable to use the advanced hand VRT techniques sparingly at a first treatment, as a more powerful application is not always necessary to achieve results. It is also best to introduce advanced techniques at the end of a session when the person is relaxed and you have ascertained verbally, and through the hands, exactly what key reflexes need working. All the techniques in this chapter can be applied to the weight-bearing hands, and most can also be applied to the passive hands. They can all be adapted for self-help.

Advanced VRT hand techniques covered in this chapter

- **Stimulation of neural pathway reflexes and incorporating Zonal Triggers** Working specifically with knuckles on the spinal reflexes and stimulating three reflexes simultaneously on the hand for a priority condition.

- **Fingertip Pressure** A unique way of working the weight-bearing fingers that is particularly helpful for head, neck or sinus conditions.

- **Palmar Pressure technique** Weight-bearing on the ball of the hand primarily for orthopaedic and digestive conditions.

- **Knuckle Dusting** Stimulation of the central nervous system and general toning techniques.

- **Palming** A stimulating technique that is gentler than Knuckle Dusting but complementary to it.

- **Lymphatic Stimulation** Basic Lymphatic Stimulation is the final new technique to be learnt in this chapter. It is a simplified version of a treatment devised by my Belgian colleague, Hedwige Dirkx.

Combinations for advanced hand techniques

There are three ways of incorporating the combined Basic and Advanced VRT techniques into the following treatments:

- **First aid** Advanced techniques are applied to the hands in an emergency situation after the body has been swiftly primed by applying the opening basic VRT techniques on the wrists and spinal reflexes.

- **Five-minute VRT treatment** Apply the basic VRT for two to three minutes, then select various advanced techniques and finish with the Harmoniser. Ideally conclude with two minutes of Diaphragm Rocking.

- **Standard VRT/reflexology hand treatment** A conventional hand reflexology treatment takes 30 to 35 minutes, and up to a total of ten minutes of VRT can be added onto or incorporated into the session. This reduction does not compromise the efficacy of the treatment, as the VRT techniques themselves are so powerful.

Stimulation of the neural pathways and Zonal Triggers

The body functions smoothly and healthily when the central nervous system is working well. The function of this system is to relay information to and from the brain from all parts of the body (see Chapter 8). It is said that about 50 per cent of all health problems are related to spinal disorders or misalignment, and these problems do not just manifest themselves in painful back conditions. The spinal

---

PRACTITIONER'S CASE STUDY

Condition: Paralysis of left side caused by a stroke.
Client: Male. **Aged:** 65.
Duration of illness: Six years.
Aim of treatment: To improve mobility.
Result: Eleven conventional reflexology treatments produced a slow improvement. After beginning VRT, the improvement was immediate and remarkable.
Practitioner's comment: Before the VRT treatments began the client had improved from being in a wheelchair to shuffling unaided and driving his car. After only two VRT sessions, as well as a full reflexology treatment, he could walk instead of shuffling – to the point where his wife asked him to slow down! He continues to come for treatment and is amazed at his accelerated progress.
Author's comment: The body has an amazing ability for regeneration given the correct impetus. Many carers of stroke patients can learn the basic VRT techniques that will help aid recovery in between professional treatments.

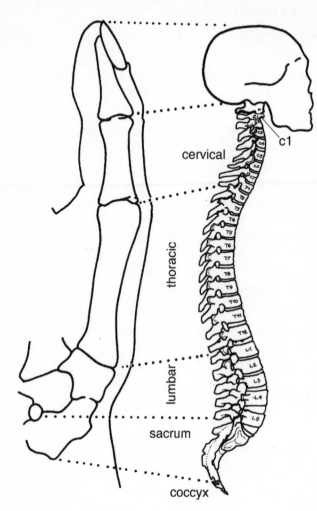

Blood supply to...

C1 Pituitary gland, brain, facial nerves, inner & outer ear

C2 Eyes, sinuses, optical & auditory nerves, tongue

C3 Outer ear, cheeks, teeth, trifacial nerve

C4 Eustacian tube, centre face

C5 Vocal cords, neck glands

C6 Shoulders, neck muscles, tonsils

C7 Thyroid, elbows

T1 Fore-arms, wrists, hands & fingers, oesophagus

T2 Cardiac system

T3 Respiratory system, breasts & chest

T4 Gall bladder

T5 Liver, solar plexus

T6 Stomach

T7 Pancreas, duodenum

T8 Spleen, diaphragm

T9 Adrenals

T10 Kidneys

T11 Ureters, kidneys

T12 Small intestines, lymph

L1 Colon

L2 Abdomen, upper leg, appendix

L3 Reproductive system, bladder, knee

L4 Prostate gland, sciatic nerve, muscles of the lower back

L5 Lower legs, ankles feet and toes

SACRUM Hip bones, buttocks, bladder

COCCYX Rectum, anus

The spinal and neural pathway reflexes in relation to the thumb

The Nervous System is extremely complex. This chart offers simplified guidelines for reflexologists and indicates links between the spinal vertebrae and some nerve inervations to various parts of the body. It does not purport to be a precise medical chart. Parts of the body are supplied by different sets of nerves such as the sympathetic and parasympathetic nervous systems and these nerves can stem from various parts of the spinal cord. The reflexologist can still work effectively when using VRT to stimulate the neural pathway reflexes by using the techniques described in this chapter. Results can be obtained by locating the distinct *pinprick* sensation on reflexes when a connection is made between the appropriate Zonal Trigger, nerve and body reflexes.

column protects the spinal cord from which an extensive array of nerves extend to specific parts of the body. If the spine is compromised in some way then the central nervous system's functions are also impaired. The aim of this technique is to fine-tune the working of the 31 pairs of cervical and spinal reflexes by simultaneously working the appropriate spinal vertebra reflex, each of which also contains a spinal nerve reflex, and the corresponding organ reflex on the hand. The vertebrae numbers should be considered as reflexes. For example, when working the shoulder reflex, refer to the chart and then work C6 at the base of the thumb, which is the shoulder neural pathway reflex. (Refer to the chart of the central nervous system and corresponding vertebrae on the left which indicates some of the main links between the vertebrae and nerve innervations.)

This technique can also be used on a client who is in the reclining position and whose hands are not weight-bearing although the results are less powerful. The working of the actual dorsal reflex and the Zonal Trigger are the same, but instead of finding the corresponding reflex on the foot or hand as in basic VRT, locate the powerful corresponding neural pathway reflex on the same hand.

For the best results it is important to use the side of your knuckle, or the outer side or edge of your thumb, and work down the medial (inside) spinal reflexes until you come to the appropriate reflex area. The use of the knuckles on the metacarpal bone spinal reflexes allows you to work deep into these reflexes where the neural pathway reflexes are located. This is called working 'bone-on-bone'. The cervical vertebrae reflexes start just below the medial thumbnail, and the lumbar, sacral and coccyx reflexes are situated just above the wrist. The key to finding the correct neural pathway reflex is when the client reports a distinct pinprick sensation. When treating the spine itself you will need to work the secondary set of spinal reflexes situated on the lateral (outer) side of the dorsum (top of the hand), which leaves the medial neural pathway reflexes free to be worked bone-on-bone. In this case the Zonal Trigger is located on the lateral side of the hand.

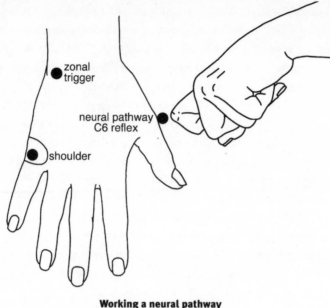

zonal
trigger

neural pathway
C6 reflex

shoulder

Working a neural pathway

When the neural pathways, including the appropriate Zonal Trigger, are stimulated, the third reflex worked is a spinal hand reflex, rather than the actual foot reflex used in standard synergistic reflexology or Zonal Trigger stimulation (see Chapter 3). When two or three reflexes are linked to the neural pathway points there can be a pulsating sensation in one or more of the reflex points. The therapist and/or the client can sometimes feel the pulses change as the various reflexes respond more powerfully at different times as the body balances. For example, the dorsal shoulder reflex and Zonal Trigger are worked with one hand and the neural pathway reflex C6 is simultaneously worked with the index knuckle of your other hand (see the illustration above).

> The neural pathway techniques described below
> are extremely powerful and beneficial when used in
> conjunction with the VRT nail-working techniques
> in Chapter 5.

Method

After basic VRT you will have ascertained the priority reflex that needs stimulating with the neural pathway reflex and the Zonal Trigger. While the client is reclining or has their hand in the passive position you will be able to work several neural pathway combinations as the effects are more subtle when the hands are not weight-bearing. These reflexes are much easier to locate when the hand is weight-bearing.

1. Briefly brush and press the reflexes around the wrists for a few seconds to activate the energy to the zones.

2. Find the specific priority reflex on the dorsum (top) of the hand and work it briefly.

3. In the usual way locate and work the Zonal Trigger simultaneously with the selected reflex point using your thumb and one finger. If you are treating the spine itself you must use the lateral helper spine and corresponding Zonal Trigger, which leaves the medial (inside) side of the hand free to locate the appropriate neural pathway.

4. With your other hand, locate the appropriate neural pathway/spinal reflex with your knuckle, or side of the thumb, and work it firmly. The reflex may feel very sharp or painful. Consult the chart on page 60 to find the approximate location of the neural pathway reflex and work precisely up and down this small area until the client reports a pinprick sensation.

5. Briefly stimulate all three reflexes simultaneously and then hold the three for a maximum of 30 seconds. Repeat on the other hand. If the problem is a right- or left-sided condition only, it is still imperative that you treat the corresponding shadow areas of the three reflexes on the other hand.

PRACTITIONER'S CASE STUDY

Condition: Frozen shoulder.

Client: Female. **Aged:** 53.

Duration of illness: Five months.

Aim of treatment: To improve mobility in the shoulder and alleviate the pain following unsuccessful keyhole surgery. The client received physiotherapy at the same time.

Result: Instant improvement in mobility after basic VRT and Zonal Trigger/neural pathway techniques. Within three treatments, over a period of eight days, the client could raise her arm almost vertically, and is now able to raise it forwards in a lateral position.

Practitioner's comment: Diaphragm Rocking, Lymphatic Stimulation, Knuckle Dusting and the Harmoniser were used, as well as lots of relaxation techniques. The client could also reach her waist comfortably and touch her ear. She also exercised her shoulder as advised by the physiotherapist, but it seemed that reflexology helped this remarkable progress the most.

Author's comment: This is an interesting example of how VRT/reflexology can help to heal an intransigent problem. Despite surgery and physiotherapy the client had very restricted movement and pain before VRT was applied.

Manual Neuro-Therapy – nerve reflexology on the spinal reflexes

There is a more medical approach to stimulating the nerve reflexes which is a technically complex, but extremely effective way of treating the body. Reflexologists find that a modified version called Manual Neuro-Therapy can enhance all treatments including VRT.

The techniques were devised by a German reflexologist, Walter Froneberg, in the 1960s, and developed for physiotherapists by Nico Pauly, a Belgian physiotherapist. Manual Neuro-Therapy locates a number of nerve reflex points on the foot skeleton. Pressing these points can rebalance the disturbed stimulus–response reactions within a few seconds. This form of therapy combines three techniques closely related to each other: neuro-muscular massage, manipulation of the spine, and neuro-reflexology. Manual Neuro-Therapy can only be taught to physiotherapists, osteopaths and chiropractors, but neuro-reflexology can be used by any well-trained reflexologist who attends an intensive postgraduate course on the topic (see Useful Addresses, page 191).

Finger-pressure technique

This VRT technique, where the fingers are individually weight-bearing, appears to be successful in treating sensitive head and neck reflexes. Conditions that particularly benefit from this technique are headaches, sinus and ear problems, eye conditions and lack of neck mobility.

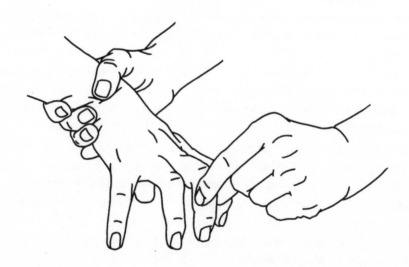

Finger-pressure technique

Method

Never treat the palm of the hand in this position as the tendons are taut and could be damaged by excess pressure.

1. The client places their right thumb and fingertips in a crab-like position firmly on a flat surface, ensuring that the hand is weight-bearing, but only enough to cause subtle pressure on the fingers.

2. Swiftly work around the base of the thumb and each finger to loosen and stimulate the cervical reflexes. Repeat on the other hand.

3. Using your thumb and index finger, starting from the base, pinch down the lateral (outside) and medial (inside) sides of the client's thumb in small bites to ensure that all the reflexes are worked. Immediately return to the base and repeat the procedure by pinching the palm and dorsal (top) sides of the thumb from the base to the thumbnail.

4. Repeat on the four fingers one by one.

- You have the option of just working one finger or thumb on each hand if you have already located a precise reflex you wish to treat.

- Repeat this sequence on the left hand.

- Always remember to work the same area of reflexes on both hands even if the problem is one-sided.

PRACTITIONER CASE STUDY

A London VRT practitioner worked on a male client who had severe Multiple Sclerosis (MS) and was confined to a wheelchair. He was incontinent and unable to move his left hand and could not grip with his right. She began giving him VRT treatments including work on the neural pathway reflexes. Within four months he had complete bladder control, his fingers started to move and he could grip with both hands. He moved away but kept in touch with the reflexologist – he has assured her that although he is still wheelchair-bound, he is very well and can stand without assistance.

There are no claims made that VRT can cure chronic disease but, in the case of MS, we have many reports that the VRT/reflexology treatments have helped to dissipate some of the symptoms.

Palmar Pressure technique

The metacarpal bones are the longest bones in the hands and form the centre of the hand. The Palmar Pressure technique takes pressure on the weight-bearing hand one stage further as only the ball of the hand is placed on the table, leaving the back of the hand slightly arched. The extra pressure placed on the spinal and other reflexes appears to give more stimulation to specific reflexes. It is particularly useful for helping digestive, sinus, neck, shoulder and back problems. Palmar Pressure, when used on the lateral abdominal organ reflexes, creates an unusual three-dimensional access as they can be worked from both sides at once. The unique benefit of Palmar Pressure (and Metatarsal Pressure and Plantar Stepping on the feet) is that the palm or sole reflexes, which are usually inaccessible with VRT, can be reached while the hand or foot is still weight-bearing.

Method

The client places their right hand on the table and presses firmly down on the top part of the metacarpal bones where they are wider and form the ball of the hand near the base of the fingers. The base of the hand is pulled upwards (approximately 45 degrees) revealing the lower part of the palm. This position is beneficial for treating certain reflexes but it is not a comfortable position and should be used only occasionally to specifically treat a particular reflex.

1. Work firmly along the spinal reflexes ending at the axle/axis reflex on the thumb adjacent to the nail. Support the client's thumb with your other hand.

2. You can gently support the bent hand by placing your hand underneath the lower palm. Continue to work down the length of the spinal reflexes to the heel of the hand.

3. Always work both hands to balance. The positive results obtained do not always seem to depend on the actual pressure but more on the angle of the hand, which appears to make deeper spinal and abdominal reflexes more accessible.

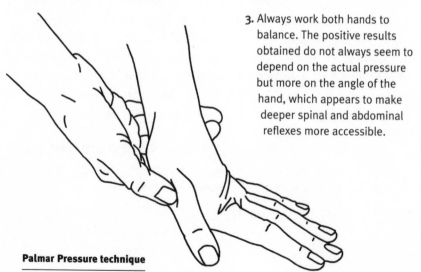

Palmar Pressure technique

Knuckle Dusting

Knuckle Dusting is an unusual method based on sweeping movements with the knuckles on the top of a weight-bearing hand. It appears to have a stimulating effect on the central nervous system – possibly by triggering a response from the thousands of tiny nerve reflexes that spread out from the spinal cord reflexes to the various organs. This is an extremely powerful technique and should be limited to about 15 to 20 seconds per hand. It can be very helpful for conditions as diverse as asthma, neck and shoulder problems and depression, and can be followed by the Palming technique.

Method

This technique should be lightly administered so the knuckles just brush the surface.

1. With a straight arm make your hand into a fist with the thumb either tucked under or loosely sticking out at its natural angle.

2. Place your fist downwards onto the client's hand and flick your wrist so that both sets of knuckles on your hand alternately touch and skim the entire dorsal (top) surface in a rolling, repetitive and twisting movement.

3. The general outcome is an invigorating effect on the body and may cause a momentary feeling of light-headedness – so ensure that there is always a table or chair available for support if the client is not already sitting down.

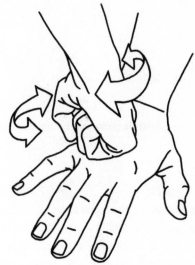

Knuckle Dusting technique

Palming

Palming stimulates the body by using the heel of the hand on the entire dorsal (top) area. It is not a means of massaging the hands but rather the application of firm pressure in a specific sweeping/twisting movement; it can be practised for up to 30 seconds on each hand.

Method

The therapist works the client's left hand with their right hand and then vice versa. Your fingers must be free to pivot around approximately 180 degrees using the lateral (outside) edge of your palm at wrist level.

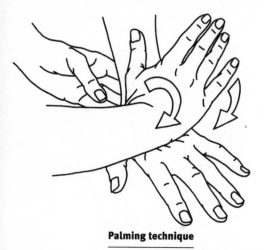

Palming technique

1. Place your left hand on top of the client's weight-bearing right hand and tilt your wrist approximately 45 degrees so that your fingers are pointing upwards.

2. Use the edge of the lateral heel of your palm, just above the wrist, to make short, rolling, twisting clockwise motions over the entire top of the hand.

3. When you touch sensitive reflexes, work them again. This method of targeting the Palming technique is particularly helpful when working the shoulder reflexes, as the lateral edge of the hand can become very sensitive with experience.

A cautionary tale

An enthusiastic reflexologist treated a new client who complained of a recurrent back injury. She immediately applied advanced VRT techniques before he had even reclined in the chair. His lower lumbar spinal reflexes felt particularly tender as she worked the priority reflexes for one minute each – she had forgotten the VRT rule is 30 seconds maximum. The client almost fainted but then revived within a minute and declared his backache had completely gone. He was delighted with the end result and sent colleagues to see her. The reflexologist, however, was very concerned as she wanted the same spectacular results but with less drama. My advice was to offer a new client a few minutes of basic VRT on arrival. Leave advanced techniques until the end of the session. Never work a reflex for more than 30 seconds. Always use the Harmoniser technique at the end of each treatment.

Lymphatic Stimulation

The body's lymphatic system is a drainage system for the circulation and the lymph nodes, which play an important part in removing toxins from the body and increasing the immunity. Lymphatic Stimulation is a very useful technique for restoring balance to this system. Lymphatic Stimulation can be used in its own right or before Diaphragm Rocking and can be applied for up to two minutes per hand. Lymphatic Stimulation and Diaphragm Rocking are not standard VRT techniques but are complementary reflexology methods I have devised to use on the passive hands. Lymphatic Stimulation is a simplified form of the Dirkx Method of Lymphatic Stimulation, which is more complex and was developed by my VRT tutor, Hedwige Dirkx.

Method

The aim of Lymphatic Stimulation is to work your client's hands simultaneously in a sweeping movement to the outside or lateral part of the hand.

The client places their elbows on a cushion and holds their palm outwards towards the therapist with their fingers facing downwards. Ideally you will work both hands simultaneously in the same way you would apply Lymphatic Stimulation to the feet. You may find it slightly more awkward to work the hands so practise first on one hand at a time until you are fully proficient.

1. Place one of your thumbs on the solar plexus reflex of each hand. Your hands will be comfortably turned so that your thumbnails are pointing towards their fingers.

2. Press your thumbs firmly on the palms on the line of the diaphragm below the middle finger, and in a sweeping movement make an arch with your thumbs across all the abdominal reflexes, ending in the area of the medial lumbar spine.

3. Repeat these movements five times so that the thumbs start a little further along the diaphragm reflexes of the spine. Ensure you press firmly on the bladder reflex on the fourth or fifth pass to stimulate the process of elimination of toxins and excess fluid, and to increase the flow of lymphatic fluid.

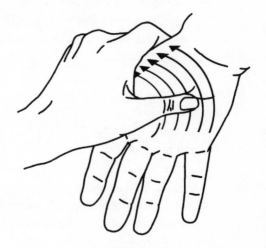

Each movement stimulates the reflexes that affect the abdominal organs and the sweeping movements are designed to help cleanse the body.

Lymphatic Stimulation

Incorporating advanced VRT techniques into a session

Now that you have learnt the advanced VRT techniques we can explore how to incorporate them into a reflexology session.

Complete hand VRT

Complete hand VRT is an option that many reflexologists use as they seek new ways to improve their services to clients. The client receives a 15- to 25-minute treatment where conventional hand reflexology is sandwiched between VRT at the start and finish of the treatment. Complete hand VRT offers a shorter treatment than the 30 to 35 minutes that is considered standard in most practices. Because VRT is so powerful as a therapy, and many results can be obtained within five minutes, the client will still receive an adequate amount of treatment to bring about benefits even though the treatment time is slightly curtailed. Because of the shortened treatment time, it is ideal for use in the workplace, for treating groups of people such as sports teams, for children and for the elderly who are unable to cope with longer sessions. The actual duration of the treatment can be flexible according to the client and therapist's wishes:

- The client receives up to five minutes of basic VRT hand treatment on arrival.

- The therapist and client then sit down or the client reclines on a couch and conventional hand reflexology is applied to the hands for approximately ten minutes. The work is mainly on the palms as the dorsum (top) of the hands will have been fully worked during the commencement of VRT.

- Halfway through the conventional treatment, the Body Brush, Lymphatic Stimulation and Diaphragm Rocking can be sequentially applied to both hands, that is, apply specific techniques to both hands.

- At the end of the treatment the wrists and spinal reflexes are swiftly worked and then some advanced and nail-working techniques should be applied according to the assessment of the condition.

- The treatment concludes with the Harmoniser technique to consolidate the work, and the client is shown a few reflex points on the hands to work daily between professional appointments to accelerate the healing processes.

Many therapists query how such a short treatment can be effective and some feel that the client is compromised by not having a full session during which they can rest and relax as they are treated. My feeling is that a 30- to 35-minute reflexology treatment for the hands and a 50- to 60-minute treatment for the feet is the ideal way for a client to relax and have space and time to themselves. However, for many people this is not a practical option for the following reasons – this is where the highly effective and shorter VRT treatments come into their own:

- The client cannot afford the cost of a full hour or extended hand reflexology treatment.

- An employee in a workplace cannot take much time during the working day to be treated.

- An employer cannot spare a member of staff for more than half an hour but is willing to subsidise their VRT treatment or, if the employee pays, they allow them paid time off during the working day to attend.

- The chronically sick and elderly in hospitals, residential homes and hospices are not able to sustain a treatment for more than 20 to 30 minutes.

- Children are often very happy to have a 15- to 30-minute treatment but would become distracted if it continued for longer.

- Many reflexologists now treat sports teams and will be booked for, say, a three-hour session. Within that time they can offer a variety of treatments depending on need. This could range from a five-minute basic hand VRT treatment for a twisted ankle to half an hour for a long-term chronic groin injury. The flexibility of complete VRT on the hands and feet allows the therapist the freedom to vary the length of treatment according to need.

- Reflexologists and interested readers particularly welcome the scope of complete VRT when it comes to treating family and friends. Many partners, including my own, complain that they do not get treated very often. This is because a therapist is not at their most enthusiastic or willing to treat the family late at night after a long day's work! Now, with a clear conscience, you can offer an extremely effective 20-minute treatment complete with Diaphragm Rocking to help any condition and provide the person you are treating with deep, peaceful sleep.

VRT and long-term healing

I was concerned in the early days of VRT that some of the newly mobile residents at my nursing home clinic would suffer wear and tear on their joints as, after treatment, they were walking further than normal, and climbing stairs. Some form of regeneration or remission must occur with VRT because many people treated by myself and colleagues over seven years ago have still maintained that flexibility with no ill effect.

Variations on the complete VRT treatment

When using VRT in a complete treatment the same options apply as in a full reflexology session – it depends on the preference of each reflexologist.

Mode 1

Hand VRT is applied for a maximum of five minutes at the beginning and end of a complete VRT session, as well as Body Brush, Lymphatic Stimulation and Diaphragm Rocking mid-point. At the end of the treatment the wrists and spinal reflexes are quickly worked, then synergistic reflexology, Zonal Trigger, and advanced techniques are applied at the end for up to five minutes.

Reason for this mode of treatment This is my preferred method of treatment as the basic VRT at the beginning gives me information about the client as well as stimulating and working the body before they lie down. At the end of the treatment I have all the information I need to work specifically on certain reflexes using the advanced VRT techniques.

Mode 2

Use basic VRT for one to three minutes at the beginning of a session and include the synergistic reflexology and Zonal Trigger work at the same time as well as a few other advanced techniques. Body Brush, Diaphragm Rocking and Lymphatic Stimulation are always used mid-point. No VRT is applied at the end of the session.

Reason for this mode of treatment The client is too relaxed to want to stand at the end of a session, or has to hurry off immediately the treatment is concluded, or the therapist wants to stimulate the body first so that it responds better to conventional reflexology. For a first treatment advanced VRT techniques are not advised at the commencement of a session, as the therapist has no knowledge of the sensitivity of the client – or how they will react to the treatment.

Mode 3

Use basic VRT at the end of a session and include synergistic reflexology, Zonal Trigger and advanced techniques. Body Brush, Diaphragm Rocking and Lymphatic Stimulation are always used mid-point. No VRT is applied at the beginning of the session.

Reason for this mode of treatment The client needs to be made comfortable at once and does not want to stand for VRT on arrival. Also you need to find out which reflexes are a priority before working with advanced VRT techniques.

Mode 4

Hand VRT is applied for up to five minutes at the beginning and end of a VRT treatment, as well as Body Brush, Lymphatic Stimulation and Diaphragm Rocking mid-point. At the end of the treatment the wrists and spinal reflexes are quickly worked. The weight-bearing hand and foot are then worked simultaneously while applying synergistic reflexology and Zonal Trigger work. Advanced techniques are then applied once only at the end of the treatment for about three to four minutes.

Reason for this mode of treatment This is usually used on clients with acute problems or on those who have suffered accidents and whose body is in trauma. Here you will have turned up the power of the reflex response because both the hand and foot are weight-bearing. Do not use this method for chronic cases on your first, or possibly second treatment, as you need to know how a client will respond. Their body will need a shorter and more subtle VRT treatment to allow time for gradual regeneration. Basic VRT is so powerful in its own right that often there is no need to use the deeper measures as the client will have already responded. Save this mode for the really intransigent cases.

Comment All methods produce excellent results and as VRT is so flexible and responsive I see no problem with adopting any of the above procedures. The lesson here is to be adaptable to individual needs and circumstances.

Sample VRT treatment using advanced techniques

Below is an example of how to treat a complaint using advanced VRT techniques. Select the priority reflex based on the individual condition.

Example: treating a severe cold

1. The five-minute basic VRT treatment can be given at the start of a session. At the end, some of the advanced techniques can be applied as appropriate. Simultaneously work all the fingers and thumbs in sequence backwards and forwards to clear the sinuses and make at least two passes across the lymphatic reflexes.

2. Apply the full conventional hand treatment (see Chapter 2) for approximately 20 to 25 minutes and include Body Brush, Lymphatic Stimulation and Diaphragm Rocking at the mid-point.

Response time to application of VRT techniques

It is impossible to accurately predict when a person will respond and improve following VRT and reflexology. Therapists and members of the medical profession are right to be cautious about raising hopes of recovery, as an individual's own genetic inheritance, constitution and immune system will determine how they react to various therapies or medication. VRT has been very successful in helping the body to recover, or begin to improve, very quickly. Most therapists suggest a client gives VRT/reflexology a fair trial by having a total of four to six treatments in total, weekly or twice weekly. Then their case should be reassessed.

3. At the end of the treatment the client places their hands firmly on a table or presses their weight-bearing hand down beside them onto a low table or chair.

4. Always use a brisk 15 seconds of Knuckle Dusting on both hands at the end of a treatment and, in this case, follow it with Palming on the chest/lymphatic/sinus reflexes.

5. Finger Pressure technique is essential when treating sinus problems, as the individually weight-bearing fingers contain the sinus and helper-sinus reflexes. Work up and down each finger and thumb in a pinching movement. If the client reports it is extra painful then back off, but gently rotate on the tender reflexes for a few seconds.

6. Synergistic reflexology: two other priority reflexes can be worked on the hands and feet, such as one of the tender sinus reflexes and a lymphatic reflex to boost the immune system.

7. Work three reflexes together. Find the most tender reflex on the chest/lung area and connect to a Zonal Trigger on the wrist with one hand. With your other hand stimulate the neural pathway reflexes by working the T3 chest/lung reflex (see page 60) with your knuckle. The client may report a pinprick sensation on a tender reflex.

8. Complete the treatment with the Pituitary Pinch and the Harmoniser.

> **Reminder**
> - Treat chronic conditions two to three times a week.
> - Acute conditions can be treated once or twice daily.
> - Self-help techniques can be used frequently throughout the day for acute conditions and twice a day for chronic conditions.

Enhancing VRT treatments

As you become more proficient in using VRT and the accompanying techniques, you will be able to decide which combination of methods and reflex points is most relevant for certain conditions. Sometimes a practitioner will begin to get results on a first treatment using VRT, Diaphragm Rocking and synergistic reflexology/Zonal Trigger. At other times VRT and various advanced techniques will be used but the client may still appear to have reached a plateau as far as further recovery is concerned. The VRT nail-working techniques you will learn in Chapter 5 can further enhance your treatments. The permutations are numerous – see below for some examples. Basic VRT should be used first, for between one and five minutes at the beginning or end of a session or both.

Combinations of advanced VRT techniques

Synergistic reflexology Simultaneously work the hand in a weight-bearing, rather than passive, position, as well as the standing foot. This is a very powerful combination and should not be used on the first treatment.

Zonal Triggers Work the neural pathway reflex on the spine while the hand is in the Palmar Pressure position. This is useful when helping chronic conditions.

Knuckle Dusting and Palming techniques Use on the weight-bearing hands and then immediately repeat the actions on the top of the weight-bearing feet.

Palmar Pressure The heel of the weight-bearing hand is raised from the flat surface so that more pressure is put on the upper metacarpal bones. This is a useful technique for working the cervical, spinal and some digestive reflexes. The client's hands are worked together and the therapist pinches simultaneously up and down the lateral reflexes of the hands.

Key points to remember

- Advanced VRT techniques enhance all reflexology treatments. Use them discerningly, especially on sensitive clients, and do not use them for a first treatment.

- Do not apply advanced techniques without at least working the wrist, spinal and pelvic reflexes first with VRT.

- The neural pathway reflexes are much more responsive when the knuckles or the inside edge of the thumb are used.

- Always use Palmar Pressure if there are neck, back and shoulder problems.

- With Knuckle Dusting, ensure that you work quickly and cover the entire hand with swift, twisting movements.

- When Palming, use the lateral heel of your palm so you can work smaller clusters of reflexes.

- The Fingertip Pressure technique can be taught to your clients as a basic self-help technique.

- Use the Harmoniser technique frequently especially when working on sensitive clients, or if the person treated comments on a slight reaction or sensation as you work.

Chapter 5

VRT nail-working

This chapter introduces a revolutionary new extension to reflexology, and to VRT in particular, in the form of VRT nail-working. My method combines the original VRT weight-bearing techniques already learnt with a technique to stimulate the minute grid-system of reflexes on the nails.

Reflexologists have always known that the pads of the thumbs are particularly receptive to fine-tuning techniques because most therapists follow the traditional view which suggests that each thumb or big toe-pad represents a mini-version of all five zones in the body, i.e. the five zones within zone 1. My findings when developing vertical reflexology have shown that the fingers and other toes provide back up and fine-tuning of the other four zones by offering their own grid system on each nail. I call this the secondary nail approach. Pressure on a part of the nail corresponding to a specific reflex can cause the actual reflex being worked to pulsate as it is activated. You can view it as being a tiny junction box on the thumbs, or big toes, which allows us to turn up the power and gain an energetic response between the reflexes and all parts of the body.

The basic technique of nail-working involves pressing your thumb- or fingernail tip onto the client's nail, working the grid-system, preferably when the hand is weight-bearing. The nail-on-nail technique appears to be highly stimulating to the reflexes situated below the nail, especially as these reflexes are always under the slight, weight-bearing pressure of the nail itself. The power of VRT is enhanced when the knuckles work the spinal reflexes, bone-on-bone, and the natural progression is to use the same principles when working nail-on-nail. Once the hand or foot becomes weight-bearing this sensitivity and response is greatly increased. You can achieve a feeling of general well-being for yourself or your clients by systematically working each nail following the VRT grid-system (see illustration, page 77) but for really effective treatments work the appropriate hand reflex and hold it while simultaneously pressing the corresponding reflex on the nail, nail-on-nail.

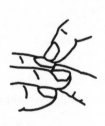

Tip of nail-on-nail

Topics covered in this chapter

- Basic VRT nail-working technique and theory.
- Treating the systems of the body with examples of the Endocrine and Digestive Flush.
- Nail-working using the secondary nail technique.
- Nail-working using the connecting knuckle technique.
- Nail-working connected to the neural pathway reflexes.

The nails on the feet and hands can be worked very effectively, and both have different merits. The great benefit of working the fingernails is that they are very accessible, larger and more uniform in shape than the toenails. The other four fingernails and the toenails represent secondary nail reflexes. The little finger-nail has a great advantage over the little toenail, which is often so small or thick-ened that it is not possible to make any

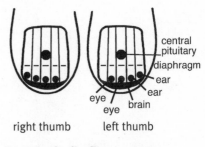

Example of nail reflexes on zones

contact other than a cursory touch with your nail tip on its centre. However, an advantage of working the toenails is that the firmer, fleshier foot makes it easier to use the knuckles to connect with the nails, specific reflexes and Zonal Triggers. The hands can be worked in the same way but the looser skin means that care must be taken to gently work the hands. Both hand and foot nail-working methods achieve equally impressive results.

Principles of nail-working for the hands (and feet)

- Every nail reflects all five zones and reflexes in half the body – see charts in Chapters 8–18. Specific nail reflexes and the corresponding hand reflex can be worked simultaneously.
- Usually the central pituitary thumb reflex only is held nail-on-nail while the dorsal reflex(es) are worked simultaneously. Holding both central pituitary nail reflexes (passive or weight-bearing) together for 30 seconds produces a sense of deep calm and relaxation.
- The eight secondary fingernails are also worked using each central pituitary reflex to connect to specific reflexes in zones 2–5. Individual reflexes can be located on all the fingernails, but not all toenails.

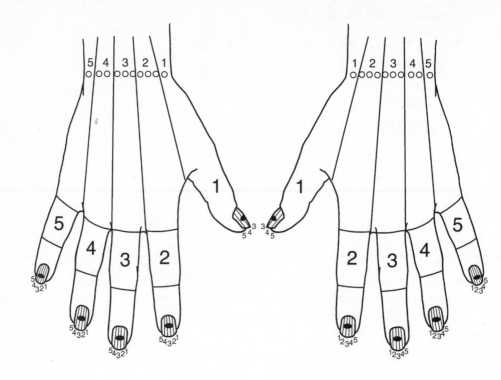

Nail and hand zones and Zonal Triggers

<table>
<tr><td>

Key point: select the VRT nail-working techniques in the same way as you would choose one of the advanced techniques.

All nails can be worked quickly or tapped vigorously to energise the body, but specific VRT nail-working should, as a general rule, be used sparingly on two or three priority reflexes at the end of a treatment.

</td><td>

Observe the grid system imposed on all the fingernails where there are five tiny rows of reflex points that mirror the zones in the body (see the illustrations above and opposite). The nails are divided in exactly the same way that the body is divided on the reflexology hand and foot charts so that in the thumb we have a tiny mirror of the larger reflex area found in the feet and hands.

</td></tr>
</table>

When to use VRT nail-working

Nail-working is an advanced reflexology technique and should usually be introduced on the second or subsequent treatments when you have ascertained the client's response to the basic VRT techniques. It takes a very different approach to Chinese finger diagnosis, with which it is occasionally confused, where the emphasis is on interpreting the colour, texture and shape of the nails to determine health status. I occasionally use nail-working when I first treat a client but I use it sparingly and would wait for the

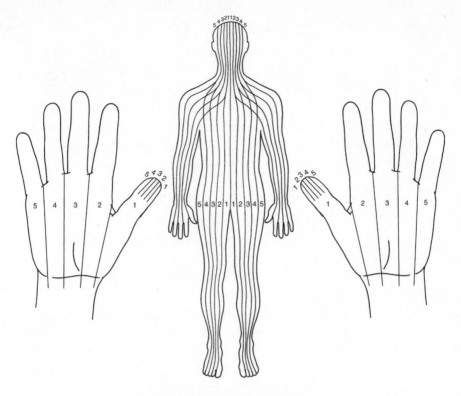

The ten reflexology zones on the body

second treatment before applying it to the nails of the chronically sick, small children or the elderly. All the nail reflexes can be treated quickly in a general way during a VRT treatment using the nail pinching relaxation techniques described in Chapter 2 or the general nail tapping described below. The various methods described in this chapter are used precisely to target and treat a few key reflexes and are another tool to add to your selection of techniques. Nail-working is excellent for self-help too.

Tapping nail-on-nail

This is a simple and useful technique to use at any time, on the passive or weight-bearing hands, as it stimulates all the reflexes within the body and can be energising. It can be used as a self-help technique or can be administered by the therapist. Simply tap, nail-on-nail, in a vigorous and random manner over all the nails on each hand for approximately 30 to 45 seconds per hand. Consider it as an additional relaxation or stimulation technique, as the body appears to respond according to its current requirements.

Self-help VRT nail-working

Self-help VRT nail-working enhances both conventional and VRT treatments, and clients can be taught to use these techniques to aid recovery in between treatments or for first-aid purposes. A useful alternative to boost your immune system is to operate a gentle, systematic pinching pressure up and down the zones of the nails and pads of your fingers, which can have a similar effect on the body as the full weight-bearing techniques. With experience, this can provide an enhanced feedback mechanism via tender or sensitised reflexes: see Chapter 6.

Applied VRT nail-working techniques

All systems and parts of the body can be accessed and can benefit from the VRT nail-on-nail techniques. To illustrate these precise techniques the endocrine and digestive systems will be used as a model.

The endocrine reflexes are particularly useful in illustrating VRT nail-work as the various reflexes cover the thumbs, the dorsum (top)/ metacarpal areas and sides of the hands as well as the wrists. Working on this area will give you a good opportunity to practise positions and movements, as various parts of the body are worked.

The central pituitary gland reflex, the master endocrine gland, appears to be contacted in an unprecedented way when the contact is made nail-on-nail, and the entire body responds.

Do I need longer nails for VRT nail-working techniques?

Absolutely not, as you will be able to very easily roll the pad of your fingertip forwards to lightly place your nail at an angle to the client's nail. The only problem would occur if the therapist bit his or her own nails down to the quick leaving just the fleshy fingertip. The reflexes under the nails on the toes and fingers are naturally subjected to more pressure when the nail itself is pressed very specifically with the therapist's own nail tip and you only need a light touch to make that important contact.

Example: treating the endocrine system – the easy option

Some therapists and readers who are keen to progress beyond the basics of VRT may well wish to use this technique first until they are more familiar with VRT nail-working methods. When working a reflex on the hand or foot you can increase the effectiveness of the treatment by connecting it to the pituitary nail reflex using the following method.

1. First place one finger or thumb on the dorsal (upper) reflex to be worked.

2. With your other hand, place your nail on the centre of the client's thumbnail (the pituitary reflex) and hold for 30 seconds. Your thumb- or finger-pad rests on the nail so you can rock your nail forwards to make intermittent contact as a pivot.

3. If desired, the dorsal reflex and Zonal Trigger can be worked simultaneously when the nail connection is made with the finger of your other hand.

4. You also have the option of making extra connections with the secondary nails by placing your nail in the centre of the fingernail, or a specific zone of a secondary fingernail that connects to a reflex in an aligned zone.

The more detailed nail reflexes and techniques below are required for a client who has not responded to these rudimentary techniques.

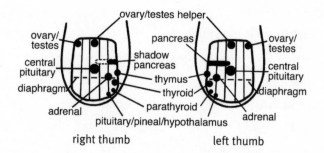

Endocrine and additional nail reflexes

Nail-working the hands individually

Method

Any system in the body can be treated in this way; just work the reflexes in sequence starting from the finger- and thumb-tips. Most importantly, you can also work individual reflexes this way.

1. On the weight-bearing hand begin by briefly working around the wrists, Zonal Triggers and the spinal reflexes down the wrists and side of the thumb in the usual manner to make the body more receptive as described in the basic hand VRT section in Chapter 3.

2. The pituitary, pineal and hypothalamus reflexes are generally considered to be in the middle of the thumb under the nail: I also work them near the medial (inside) side of the thumb. With VRT the aim is to simultaneously access each of the client's central pituitary reflexes with your finger- or thumbnails and hold for 30 seconds at the beginning of a treatment.

3. Once you have made contact with the master gland reflexes on both thumbnails, you can move swiftly down each hand, separately working each dorsal endocrine reflex in turn while you continuously exert pressure on the pituitary reflex with your nail. See the illustration on page 152 for endocrine reflexes on the hand.

The sequence is:

- First press both the pituitary reflexes simultaneously for 30 seconds nail-on-nail to stimulate and centre the body. Continue to press the right pituitary reflex.

- When working the thymus reflex only, it is easier to stimulate the reflex situated on the medial side of the client's hand with your knuckle.

- As you work down the hand (using thumb, finger or knuckles) make rotating movements on each endocrine reflex in turn and then hold for up to 10 seconds. During this sequence you or your client may become aware that a particular reflex becomes more tender or receptive, which may be due to a possible imbalance.

- Work the following:

  the thyroid and helper-thyroid

  the thymus – use your knuckle to stimulate this reflex

  the adrenal

  the pancreas

  the ovary/testes

  the helper ovary/testes

  the uterus/prostate (this is not an endocrine reflex but is influenced by the system)

- At completion apply the Harmoniser to balance the body. Repeat on the other hand.

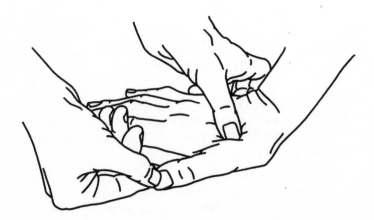

Working the adrenal reflex while holding the pituitary

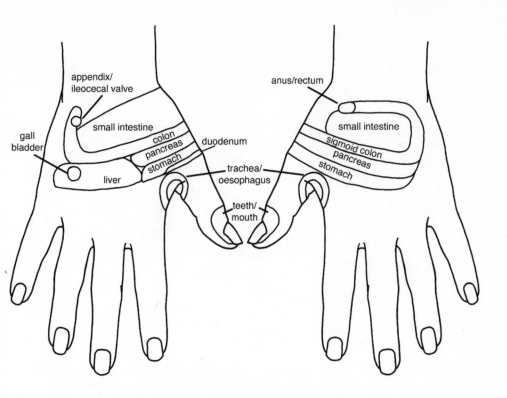

Digestive reflexes on the hand

Nail-working the hands simultaneously

This is a variation of the standard treatment and is as effective as the basic VRT nail-work treatment just described. The difference is that here the initial simultaneous nail-work on the pituitary reflexes triggers a powerful 30-second response from the reflexes to the entire body, not just the endocrine system. The stimulation of each reflex is doubled by working both hands simultaneously in sequence, starting from the teeth/mouth reflexes and ending on the rectum/anus reflexes.

The VRT flush – the digestive system

It is important to face the client, standing either side of a small table, or across a corner, so you have clear access to the top of both their weight-bearing hands.

The client sits and places their hands forwards on a low table and the therapist kneels on a cushion in front of them and works their weight-bearing hands. The therapist can also sit using a small, sloping stool that stands about 15 cm off the ground.

Method

Work the weight-bearing wrists briefly, then simultaneously press the two pituitary reflexes for 30 seconds with your nails on the weight-bearing hands as described in the nail-working method above. This is the only nail-on-nail contact in this sequence.

Simultaneously work down both hands using your index-finger-pads to stimulate all other digestive reflexes from the teeth/mouth to the anus/rectum area with your fingertips. You may use a minute amount of cream if preferred. Stimulate and then hold each set of reflexes for 10–15 seconds and then release.

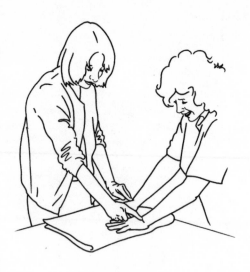

VRT treatment across a table

1. Hold the pituitary reflexes simultaneously for 30 seconds nail-on-nail, then move on to stimulate and rotate on each of the following reflexes simultaneously on both hands:

   ● the teeth/mouth reflexes

   ● the trachea/oesophagus reflexes

   ● the liver/gall bladder reflexes on the right hand and the corresponding shadow reflex area on the left

   ● the pancreas and stomach reflexes

   ● the small intestine and colon reflexes

   ● the appendix/ileocecal reflexes on the right hand and the corresponding shadow area on the left hand

   ● the rectum/anus reflexes on the left hand and corresponding area on the right

2. Use the Harmoniser to finish.

VRT connecting treatment

This method uses thumbnail reflexes connected with Zonal Triggers as well as the secondary nail treatment. The connecting nail-working techniques below offer another powerful technique to consolidate your work. As you work down the sequence of endocrine reflexes one, or possibly two, points may seem particularly tender – this can indicate an imbalance. Use your knuckle to slide down the hand; gently work the whole zone starting at the wrist, passing through the priority dorsal (upper) reflex and ending on the appropriate nail. This particular technique is easier to apply to the feet but is equally effective on the hands. If you have a problem connecting a certain priority reflex on the hand because of the thin, loose skin, try the same technique on the standing foot (see the illustration on page 88).

Balance the body

Always work both hands in exactly the same shadow areas to balance the body – even if you are treating a one-sided problem such as a shoulder, heart or liver. VRT appears to free up the entire zone and the body can feel very unbalanced if the corresponding zone is not cleared and stimulated during a treatment.

Method

For intransigent problems up to two reflexes within the same system can be prioritised for the connecting nail techniques.

During the VRT endocrine connecting treatment sequence, or when working any other system in the body, up to two reflexes can be worked with the Zonal Triggers in the following way using the Secondary Nail technique. This advanced way of working allows you to use this technique twice within the same system.

Practice example

After completing your full VRT hand and conventional treatment you will have prioritised the key reflexes to be worked. You may have already performed other advanced VRT techniques. At this point proceed as follows. This example uses the pancreas reflex as the priority reflex, as it is part of the endocrine and digestive system.

1. Return to the pituitary reflex on your client's left hand, press nail-on-nail with your thumbnail or fingernail and hold while you connect to another endocrine reflex, in this case the pancreas, which may have been the most tender reflex during the treatment.

2. Having located the specific part of the reflex on the dorsum (top) of the hand you now need to locate the appropriate pancreas Zonal Trigger using the pinprick indicator.

3. Place your thumb and index finger of the right hand on the Zonal Trigger and dorsal (upper) pancreas reflex. With your left thumbnail work the client's nail pituitary reflex and continue to hold during the connecting stages.

4. First connecting stage: now you are ready to connect the Zonal Trigger to the pancreas by lightly sliding or pressing the knuckle of your index finger along the dorsum. A minute amount of cream is helpful for these techniques. Knuckles are more powerful but the fingertips are an acceptable alternative.

5. Second stage: continue down the hand by sliding from the pancreas reflex to the pituitary reflex on the nail. This sliding action can be applied once quite firmly and twice lightly in a stroking movement.

6. These connecting techniques are very powerful for linking reflexes in zones 1 and 2.

7. Not all reflexes will be in direct line with a nail so you may have to curve the connecting line, but only within the range of two zones (see the illustration on page 88).

8. Repeat on the other hand, then select another reflex to be worked from the same system if required.

9. Finish with the Harmoniser.

Working specific nail reflexes

These fine-tuning techniques are appropriate for all reflexes situated in zones 1 to 5.

Important points to note

Basic connecting thumb work is only applicable for zones 1 and 2 – as it is not possible to effectively run a knuckle diagonally across a hand or foot. The alternative method is to use the same connecting techniques, but this time linked to the other fingernails positioned in zones 2 to 5.

- The thumbnail has a mini-map of half the body imposed on it.
- Likewise each fingernail or toenail represents all the organs, glands and the skeletal system found in the body.
- This means you have the option to press just the centre of the nail to make a general connection, or to work the five zones on the nail precisely to find the exact location of a reflex. The nail and dorsal reflexes are then simultaneously held for 30 seconds.

Connecting reflexes and secondary nails

The following is a simple and very effective way to make a connection from a reflex to a secondary nail (see illustration on page 88).

Occasionally the client will report a tender point on the nail but more often the actual reflex being worked will emit a pulse or feel tender.

1. The client places their hands firmly on a flat surface.

2. Place your thumb- or finger-pad on the centre of each of the client's thumbnails and tilt your thumb or finger forwards so that it is supported as the tip of your nail touches their nail. Briefly press your nails on their nails to balance and centre the body. Hold for 30 seconds.

3. Locate a tender reflex on the dorsum (top) of the client's hand while weight-bearing. For this example the liver reflex is used.

4. Press the liver reflex with the pad of your index finger and work up and down the client's right thumbnail using your nail to stimulate their five zones. This should take 30 seconds at most. Locate the liver nail reflex in zone 5, which is on the little fingernail in the mid-section (see illustration on page 89).

5. Hold the tip of your nail on this point for 30 seconds while simultaneously pressing the actual liver reflex on the hand.

6. Repeat this technique on the left hand to balance the zones in the body and where necessary always work the shadow reflexes.

7. Once the third point, the Zonal Trigger, has been located these three points can be held for 30 seconds. The powerful connection can then be made by gently sliding your knuckle from the Zonal Trigger, via the reflex, to the nail in a straight line. Repeat this move a total of three times on each hand.

8. Use the Harmoniser to balance the body.

If you decide to work very precisely on the thumb or secondary nail grids, you may find that a tender point near the base of the nail in zone 5, for example, indicates a problem in the hip. The top edge of the index fingernail in zone 2 may feel tender as it connects up to an eye problem. These nail reflex positions correspond to particular parts of the body as mapped out on a conventional Ingham zone chart.

Revitalising hint

Gently pinching up and down each finger and thumb and working the five tiny zones, nail-on-nail, is a very stimulating and effective calming mini-treatment for the hands which is then reflected in the entire body. (This is fully described on page 18.)

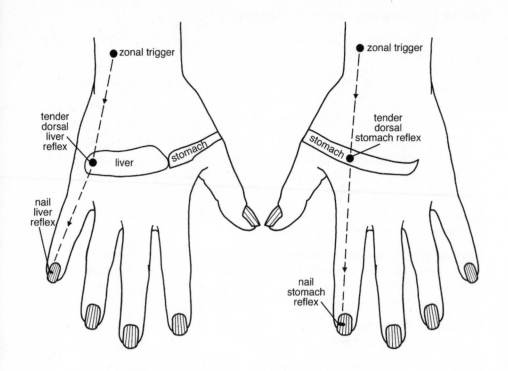

Connecting reflexes to secondary nails

Reminder when working the spinal reflexes

Always slide your fingers in as straight a line as possible from the Zonal Trigger to the nail point. The spinal reflexes will not connect directly in a straight line to the thumbnail but the helper spinal reflexes will connect as these are situated in zone 5, on the lateral (outside) side of the hand. With the thymus reflex, it is difficult to reproduce this technique because it will not connect with a nail unless you curve your knuckle up and off the side of the hand to reach the edge of the thumbnail. Throughout the procedure keep pressing nail-on-nail.

VRT nail-working and the stimulation of the neural pathways and Zonal Triggers

In Chapter 4 we covered the stimulation of the neural pathway reflexes. When connecting to a priority reflex, the neural pathway reflex on the spine is also worked in combination with the Zonal Trigger. In this chapter we go one step further by locating the priority reflex on the fingernail which is then worked with the neural pathway reflex and the corresponding Zonal Trigger. An additional

Central nervous system – brief recap

The function of the central nervous system is to relay information to and from the brain from all parts of the body (see Chapter 8). If a spinal vertebra is slightly under pressure or has been damaged in an accident, then organs and other parts of the body can be affected because the information from the nerves is inadequate. The spinal column protects the spinal cord, from which an extensive array of nerves extend to specific parts of the body. You can access the central nervous system via the medial side of the hands and feet, working down the area of the spinal points using your knuckle to precisely pinpoint a nerve reflex that corresponds to an organ, gland or part of the skeletal system.

option using a fourth reflex, the priority dorsal reflex itself, enables you to pinpoint where a reflex is situated on a nail, as the reflex may pulse when the nail reflex is located. Work the lateral spine reflexes when treating a spinal neural pathway.

Locating priority nail reflex, neural pathway and Zonal Trigger reflexes

The aim of this treatment is to find a priority reflex on the nail and link it to a corresponding Zonal Trigger and neural pathway reflex.

The method described on page 90 relies on an accurate pinpointing of the nail reflex by referring to the chart below and the response from the client when the correct neural pathway point is located (see page 60). They should be able to report a distinct pinprick sensation. This advanced technique should ideally be used at the end of a VRT treatment.

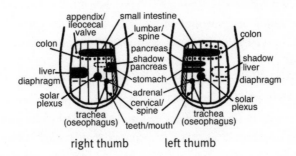

Digestive and additional nail reflexes

Working the neural pathways

1. Locate the left pancreas reflex on the thumbnail and hold it nail-on-nail while stimulating the dorsal (upper) pancreas reflex for 30 seconds.

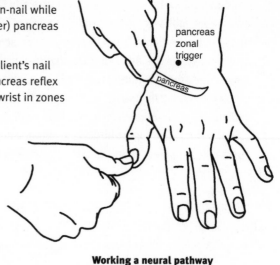

pancreas zonal trigger

pancreas

2. Remove your nail from the client's nail and return to the dorsal pancreas reflex and hold. Work around the wrist in zones 1 to 4 until you find the corresponding Zonal Trigger. Stimulate these two reflexes simultaneously for up to 30 seconds.

3. Now press a tender pancreas nail reflex, and work precisely up and down the appropriate area of the medial (inside) side of the hand with your

Working a neural pathway

knuckle until you find the neural pathway reflex that corresponds roughly to the T7 reflex where some of the main nerve innervations to the pancreas are situated (see page 60). The client should report a pinprick sensation on the nerve reflex on the medial spinal area when you have located the correct point. The reflex may occasionally throb a little and you may feel a pulsing sensation in your knuckle.

4. Hold your nail on the pancreas nail reflex while you work the corresponding neural pathway reflex as illustrated above.

5. Certain combinations of all three reflexes, including the Zonal Trigger, can very occasionally be stimulated simultaneously if you are sufficiently dexterous. Repeat on the right hand.

Summary of VRT nail-working

The actual nail-on-nail working of weight-bearing nails is a new and powerful concept that gives you extra tools with which to work. The gentle pressure of nail-on-nail is immensely powerful and calming and enables the dorsal reflexes, Zonal Triggers and neural pathway reflexes to respond much more powerfully than standard VRT techniques. The nail exercises and techniques described in this chapter, and in Chapters 8–18, can also be used to work the weight-bearing and passive hands as well as the reclining or standing feet. Nail-working is not usually a full treatment in itself but can aid you in treating intransigent problems. With the exception of the Harmoniser, which can be used straight away, nail-working should be considered from the second VRT hand treatment onwards.

Key points to remember

- A powerful but gentle treatment, nail-working involves the passive nails being worked one by one, five zones per nail. Hold the pituitary reflexes together to conclude.

- Precise targeted VRT nail-working should, as a general rule, be used sparingly on two or three priority reflexes at the end of a treatment.

- You can use the Harmoniser treatment at any time to centre and balance the body as well as at the completion.

- The endocrine system responds particularly well to VRT nail-working but every system in the body can be treated with these very powerful techniques.

- It is helpful to locate the appropriate nail reflex by first connecting it to the dorsal reflex on the hand.

- When you treat a back problem using the neural pathway connection, use the secondary helper spinal reflexes on the lateral side of the hand.

- Do not press too hard on the nails. A light touch accesses the five zones. Always support the working nail by using your thumb- or fingerpad to roll forwards until you make nail-on-nail contact.

- Good results can also be obtained by just pressing the centre of the nail and connecting with other reflexes.

Chapter 6

Self-help VRT for hands

This chapter covers the self-help aspects of hand VRT. It is useful to regularly use some of these techniques for a few minutes daily to help to maintain health or to accelerate recovery from an illness. The self-help aspects embrace all the techniques you have learnt in this book so far. Obviously you will not need to use every technique you have learnt on each treatment as it would take too long and could over-stimulate the body and cause dizziness or nausea. Instead, select suitable VRT applications from a toolbox of techniques depending on individual need.

The treatment is brief and the body responds well to work on the weight-bearing reflexes.

Reflexologists acknowledge that their therapy is far more accommodating as far as self-help is concerned than many other bodywork therapies that involve oils, needles or manipulation such as aromatherapy, acupuncture and osteopathy. With VRT the weight-bearing hands immediately become more sensitive and responsive and it is easy to work the two reflexes simultaneously on the hands and feet (see the illustration at the base of page 105) to increase the powerful response. You can even treat a priority reflex this way by working the dorsal reflex and Zonal Trigger on the foot and the corresponding dorsal reflex on the hand (see the illustration on page 106).

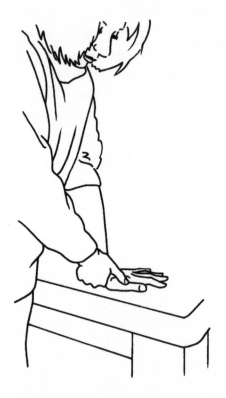

Self-help on weight-bearing hand

Introduction to the self-help hand techniques

There are four ways of treating yourself with reflexology and VRT:

Self-help hand reflexology

Treat your hands conventionally by working first one hand and then the other, using the relaxation techniques and conventional moves described here and in Chapter 2. Most VRT techniques can be applied to the passive hands.

Conventional synergistic self-help

This method combines simultaneous work on the foot and hand while seated. Three or more priority reflexes can be selected and these techniques comprise the standard concept first described in my companion book, *Vertical Reflexology*.

Self-help hand reflexology and VRT

Your hand is placed firmly on a table, palm downwards, and the basic and advanced VRT techniques are applied to the dorsum (top) of the hand, as well as the conventional hand relaxation techniques.

Weight-bearing self-help VRT and synergistic reflexology

The weight-bearing foot is placed on a chair and is worked synergistically with the hand. Advanced techniques using Zonal Triggers are applied.

VRT and synergistic reflexology appear to heighten the receptiveness in the body to the external stimulation of the reflexes. Reflexologists can treat themselves conventionally and get good results, but self-help VRT gives a more energetic response and most people report that there is greater sensitivity and a sensation similar to when one's hands are being treated by another. VRT self-help can be a major breakthrough in accelerating the healing processes as a client can be taught a few simple moves to practise twice daily in between treatment.

Learn from your clients

Carolyn was an administration manager and had suffered from intermittent back, hip and neck problems for many years. Her work was highly demanding and, at times of stress, she would become aware of muscular tension throughout her body. I advised her to work her weight-bearing hands for a few minutes, twice daily on rising and before bed, but she observed that her aches were getting worse not better. She correctly deduced that, due to her sensitivity, the amount of self-help was too powerful and she reduced it to once every other day. The result was that she rapidly improved with no ill-effects and within four to six weeks reported that she felt better than she had done for over a year.

Until then I had believed that VRT was self-regulating and could not cause an over-reaction. This was ill-advised and I now suggest caution when I teach new, sensitive or chronically ill clients the self-help hand techniques.

It is important to build up the self-help skills in a methodical manner, and even if you are a professional reflexologist it is essential to briefly treat a few reflex points on your hands in the conventional manner so that you can experience the contrasting improvement once you apply synergistic reflexology and VRT.

In your own self-help practice sessions, press firmly enough to feel a slight discomfort on areas you know to be sensitive. I do not believe in the old adage 'no gain without pain' as you can give a firm and authoritative reflexology treatment that is effective but pain-free. Always apply the Harmoniser technique, whether you work lightly or firmly.

These VRT skills will become invaluable as first-aid help when at home, at work or travelling, and you will be able to react quickly if you fall and injure yourself or perhaps feel a stomach-ache or sore throat coming on. Chronic problems can be alleviated by learning to work the appropriate reflexes for a few seconds whenever there is discomfort.

As with all VRT treatments it does not matter whether you start with the left or right hand or foot. There is only one important rule with any form of synergistic reflexology: the right hand works the right foot and the left hand works the left foot. This is to enable the energy from the stimulated hand and foot reflexes to flow through the same zone on the same side of the body.

There is one important difference when treating yourself: you do not have to keep alternating hands, as your own energy appears to keep you in balance.

Conventional self-help treatments

Begin by seating yourself comfortably in an upright chair. A bed can also be suitable if your back is supported. Place a towel-covered cushion on your lap. This allows the hand to rest comfortably and the towel will protect your clothes if you use cream. Relax the right hand first and then the left applying the appropriate relaxation techniques below. It is easier to alternate hands for each relaxation move.

Loosening the wrists

Firmly grip around your wrist with the thumb and index finger of your working hand and press firmly so that your hand feels secure. The aim is to gently shake your wrist and hand by evenly moving your working hand up and down slightly in a rocking movement while simultaneously gripping

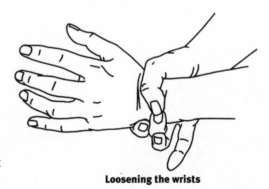

Loosening the wrists

and pinching. This is an excellent exercise for improving the circulation of the hands and preventing cold or 'dead' fingers, especially in the winter.

Squeezing the spinal reflexes

Turn the hand that is to be worked away from your body with your thumb relaxed and the palm away from you. Approaching from the medial (inside) side, place your thumb over the dorsum (top) of the hand and allow your fingers to rest on the edge of your palm. Grip and pinch the hand with your thumb and fingers as you slowly move up the hand until you reach the thumbnail. Work back down to the wrist then repeat this movement two or three times.

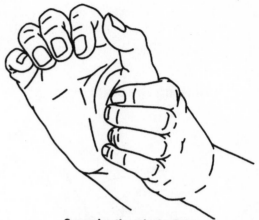

Squeezing the spinal reflexes

Whole Body Brush

Place your working hand over the dorsum (top) of your right hand with your fingertips touching the wrist bracelet and pointing in the direction of your arm. Your thumb is curved around the medial (inside) side of the hand and rests on the palm. Press your four fingers gently but firmly on the skin and move your hand towards you in tiny little bites. The whole movement should flow from the wrists to the fingertips, tenderly but firmly enough for you to be aware of the intermittent pressure as your fingers move across the top of your right hand. The movements are made three times, starting from the wrist with a firm to decreasing pressure that ends in a gentle brushing, soothing movement with your fingertips.

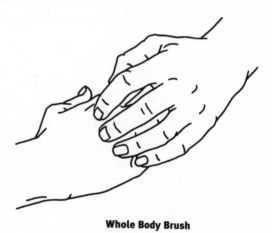

Whole Body Brush

Conventional techniques for passive hands

These techniques can be discreetly applied to your hands when travelling as a passenger, in the workplace or at any location when your body needs help but it is inappropriate or impossible for you to work the weight-bearing hands or feet. A person can be taught to work the chest/bronchial area of their hands and pinch the webbing between their thumb and fingers to help prevent a mild asthma attack. The right hand is shown being worked first for continuity.

Working the palm

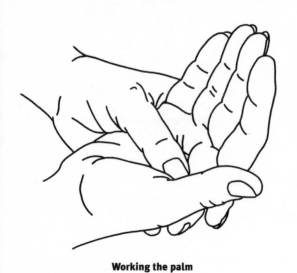

Working the palm

Use the standard reflexology thumb caterpillar technique to inch the pressure across the palm so that every reflex is stimulated. To stimulate an area of weakness work backwards and forwards in precise rotational movements on reflex areas that are tender or that correspond to a known health problem. Thirty seconds to a minute is usually enough to stimulate a reflex when using conventional reflexology on the hands.

Working the fingers and thumbs including nail-working

Use your forefinger and thumb to pinch down your fingers and thumb from the base to the nail of each finger and thumb in tiny moves or bites. This enables the head and neck reflexes to be worked on both sides at once. Work sensitively, becoming aware of any granular, hard, puffy or tender parts of the hands. Press firmly on the fingers as they contain all the head, neck, ear, eye and nose reflexes plus several endocrine glands.

Take your hand in your working hand and turn it so it is facing palm downwards. Approaching the hand from the lateral side, place your thumb underneath

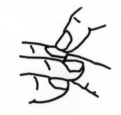

Stimulating each nail: self-help

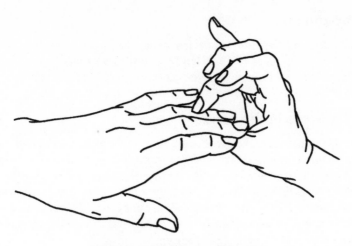

Self-help on the fingers and thumbs

your passive hand with your finger resting on the dorsum (top) of your hand. Your working index or third finger is placed on the dorsal wrist in zone 5 which aligns with the little finger. Now pinch down the side of the hand and along the little finger in small bites until your fingerpad touches your little fingernail. Arch your finger and place the tip of your fingernail at the base of the little fingernail and gently edge the tip of your fingernail along the *centre* of your nail to the tip. Repeat this move very swiftly up zones 1, 2, 4 and 5 on either side of the centre (zone 3) little finger nail grids. Repeat this entire procedure from wrist to nail on all five digits. After working three fingers (zones 5, 4 and 3) you will have to bring your working hand to the medial side of your passive hand so you can work zones 2 and then 1 (on the thumb) in the same manner. Repeat the sequence on your other hand. This can become a swift treatment with practice.

Working the webbing of the hand

Using the thumb and forefinger, pinch the webbing between your other thumb and forefinger and then between all your fingers. Your forefinger will be pinching the palm as you pull your thumb across this loose fleshy dorsal (upper) area of the hand. This boosts the immune system by stimulating the lymphatic reflexes and accesses some bronchial, eye and ear reflexes. Clients can also be taught this easy technique.

Working the webbing of the hand

Wrist-band on the hand

Press and slide your thumb across the top of the wrist several times. You can also make little caterpillar bites with your forefinger, as this will stimulate the groin, Fallopian tube, helper heart, diaphragm and Zonal Trigger reflexes.

Specific areas of the hand

- Using the guidelines in Chapter 2, swiftly run over the various systems of the body on the hands to stimulate it generally and practise a few relaxation techniques. Work each hand for between five and ten minutes, paying special attention to tender reflexes that can indicate congestion or malfunction in the body. A tender reflex does not always indicate major disease or a problem; it can show a slight imbalance. In *Hand Reflexology*, Kristine Walker suggests working the hands in specific directions as indicated on page 99.

- Once your hands have been fully worked, it is time to return to specific reflex areas that felt tender or gritty to your touch. Select three priority reflexes and work them firmly on both hands. Having located the reflexes, you would normally select one of the three reflexes as the main priority and then locate the appropriate Zonal Trigger. As you are not working the weight-bearing hands, you can locate and work all three reflexes with their corresponding Zonal Triggers, as the effect is more subtle on the body when the hand is not weight-bearing.

Example: three priority areas to be worked for practice

- adrenal glands
- neck
- stomach

These reflexes have been selected to give variety in this practice session because the adrenal glands are found on both hands, the stomach is found mainly on the left hand and the neck reflexes are situated on either side of the thumb.

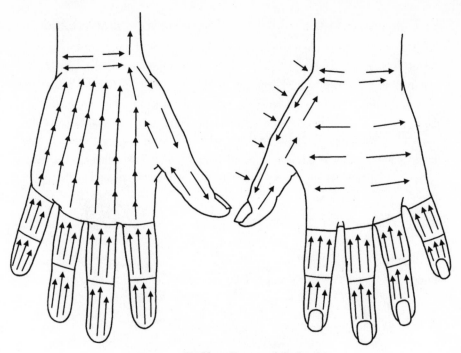

Working all areas of the hand

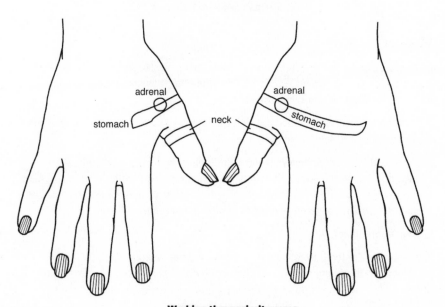

adrenal   adrenal

stomach   neck   stomach

Working three priority areas

Work each reflex in a firm rotating movement for up to a minute per reflex if the hand is not weight-bearing. Back off if it is too tender, and work gently. If the hand is weight-bearing, work reflexes for up to 30 seconds each.

VRT Harmoniser technique – self-help on the passive hand

The Harmoniser (see Chapter 3) is one of the most powerful therapeutic tools in the VRT repertoire. It incorporates nail-work on the third fingernail or toenail and is designed to prevent an over-reaction or a healing crisis following a treatment. The third zone on each hand has been chosen because it is the middle zone in the hand and can therefore act as a balancing mechanism to each side of the body. My VRT tutor, Françoise Petraman, devised the following technique that allows you to work three reflexes on one hand at once. This enhances the treatment, although the weight-bearing hand can obviously not be treated in this mode.

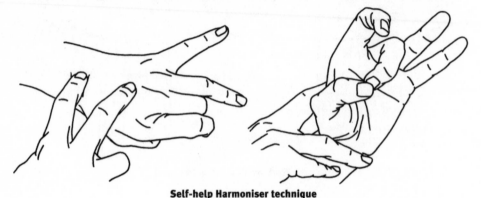

Self-help Harmoniser technique

Method

Once you have worked on your passive or weight-bearing hands and incorporated some advanced VRT techniques you should apply the following actions to consolidate the treatment and prevent over-reaction.

1. Hold up your left hand, place your left thumbnail-tip onto the centre of your third fingernail on the same hand, and hold.

2. Now simultaneously place your right third finger on the dorsal (upper) solar plexus reflex on the hand and align your right index finger with the corresponding Zonal Trigger on the wrist. Now hold all three points for 15 to 30 seconds so that you are stimulating all three reflexes in zone 3 simultaneously.

3. Repeat on the left hand.

You may also use the Harmoniser on your own weight-bearing hands by first pressing your third right nail with your third left nail. Then separately place your fingers on the dorsal Zonal Trigger and solar plexus reflexes for a few seconds.

Synergistic self-help on the passive hands

Follow the instructions on page 104 for synergistic VRT, and apply the same moves to your resting hands.

PRACTITIONER'S CASE STUDY

Condition: Baker's Cyst (behind knee).

Client: Female. **Aged:** 62.

Duration of illness: one week.

Aim of treatment: To reduce cyst and regain mobility.

Result: Cyst went down on the day of treatment and never returned.

Practitioner's comment: Client presented with Baker's Cyst, which meant she could not bend her knee or kneel. Her doctor said that the large cyst would burst. Instead it disappeared and has never returned.

Author's comments: This indicates that the reflexologist must have triggered the exact reflex connected with the cyst. Another client had a Baker's Cyst that disappeared. Whenever she feels a sensation in the back of her knee that indicates swelling, she has been taught to work the knee reflex on her hand and the sensation soon abates. I have reports of similar swift results with underarm cysts, haemorrhoids and tooth abscesses.

Self-help basic VRT treatment

Stand straight and place your right hand, palm downwards, on a table, weight-bearing downwards from your arm at all times during the treatment.

1. Slide, press or brush your thumb across the dorsal (upper) wrist.

2. Work the hip, pelvic or sciatic areas on the medial (inside) and lateral (outside) side of your hands above and below the wrists.

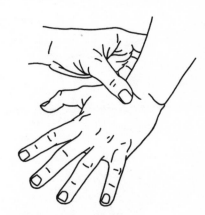

Working the wrist reflexes

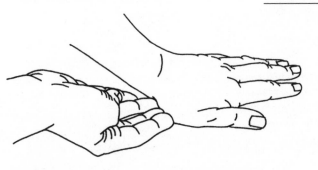

Working the medial edge of the hand: lumbar spine release

3. Move sideways to your hand. Gently press your four fingers downwards and grip the medial (inside) edge of the side of your hand below the thumb. Gently pull upwards three times.

4. For the spinal reflexes, press the vertebrae reflexes from tip of thumb to medial (inside) wrist edge with your thumb, index finger or four fingers – work the reflexes backwards and forwards three times. Tap up and down the medial side of the hand with four fingers, three times each. At this point you could proceed directly to advanced or priority techniques for a first-aid treatment.

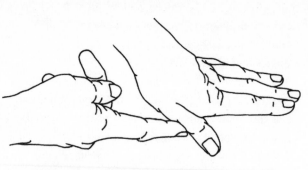

Working the medial edge of the hand: the spinal reflexes

5. Pinch twice around the lower arm circumference around the muscle for the thoracic reflexes.

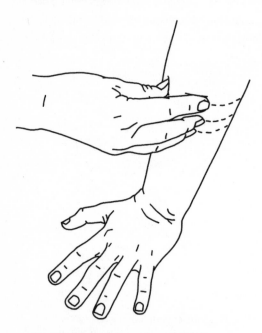

Working the lower arm: thoracic spine

6. Work your weight-bearing thumb and fingers, starting from the thumb, by making rotating movements from the base of your fingers to the tip of the nail or vice versa. Then pinch up or down the sides of the thumb and fingers in turn.

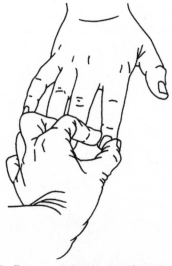

Working the fingers and thumbs: head/neck areas

7. Press the lymphatic reflexes at the base of your fingers in a rotating movement with two fingers. Work your fingers in wide circular movements to cover the metacarpal area below the bases of all the fingers and thumb.

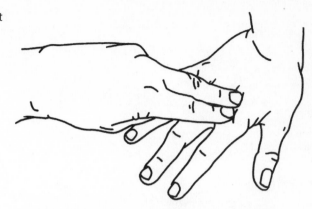

8. Return at least once to the wrist points and work these to energise the body.

Working the finger bases and metacarpal heads: lymphatic and chest reflexes

9. Press the helper ovary/testes points at the base of the heel of your hand, on the palm side as the hand presses on the table. You can also simultaneously stimulate the dorsal ovary helper reflex in a pinching movement.

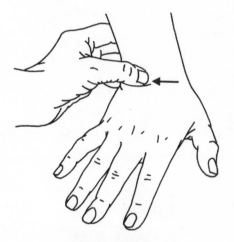

Working the helper ovary/testes reflexes

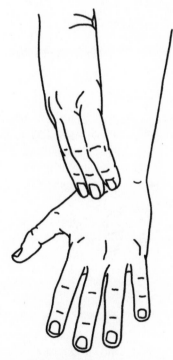

Finger-walking the metacarpals

10. Work the metacarpal area on the dorsum (top) of the hand. Stand sideways at an angle to the table and place your fingertips on the dorsal wrist and work down, in little caterpillar bites, to your fingernails. Slide off in a gliding movement. Repeat three to four times, ensuring that all the dorsal reflexes of the hand are treated.

11. Apply the Pituitary Pinch. The thumb naturally splays on its side.

12. Use the Harmoniser to finish (see instructions and illustration on page 100).

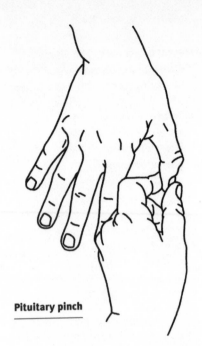

Pituitary pinch

Self-help VRT and synergistic reflexology

Synergistic reflexology is a term used to describe the working of two corresponding reflexes at the same time. In this method, the overall effect is greater than the sum of two parts, i.e. the aim of this exercise is to teach you to increase the energy to the stimulated reflexes by working the hands and the feet together.

Method

Ideally work and relax both hands as described in the conventional self-help section on the preceding pages, or apply basic VRT and self-help Diaphragm Rocking first (see page 107). During this brief treatment, ascertain up to three priority reflexes that require treatment (that is, any parts of your body that are imbalanced or malfunctioning in some way). Minor ailments, chronic illnesses and post-operative conditions may all respond to synergistic reflexology.

Having relaxed both hands, begin working again on the right hand with which you started. Remember the rule: left hand/left foot, right hand/right foot.

Synergistic VRT

Synergistic VRT can be passive, but it is better if you are physically able to stand without support and can place your foot on a chair or stair-tread.

Your body is much more receptive to reflexology once it is in a standing position, so the following sequence of techniques is the ultimate in your self-help programme. As you become more familiar with the hand reflexes you will easily adapt these basic techniques to suit your individual needs.

To experience the full VRT treatment you can follow the instructions from the basic self-help guidelines on the preceding pages. Your treatment can conclude with self-help VRT nail-working, Lymphatic Stimulation and Diaphragm Rocking as described in this chapter.

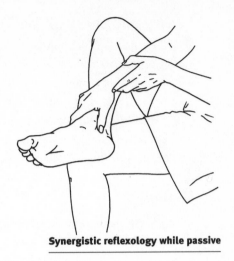

Synergistic reflexology while passive

Finding two synergistic points when self-treating

Here the kidney is used as an example.

Method

1. Place your right foot on a hard chair or stool and lean forwards so that it is weight-bearing.

2. Locate your right-hand palm kidney reflex with your left forefinger (you can work this dorsally at the same time). Maintain this position, lean forwards and place your right forefinger on the kidney reflex on the dorsum (top) of your right foot. You are now in a position to work the reflexes together, that is, your left finger works your right hand while at the same time your right hand is working the right kidney reflex. Rotate briefly and then press gently but firmly for 30 seconds.

3. You could then select one or even two more reflexes from any system in the body to work this way. It is essential to balance the body by working the same shadow reflex area on both hands and feet regardless of whether the problem is one-sided or if the organ, such as the liver, is situated on one side only.

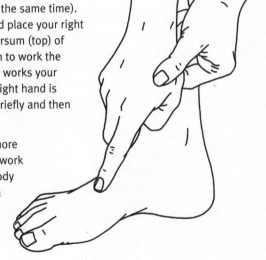

Synergistic VRT on the kidney reflex

Finding one priority Zonal Trigger while standing

When a Zonal Trigger is pressed, the body is galvanised into an extra surge of energy or rebalancing. Usually one Zonal Trigger point per treatment is worked, but once you are experienced in VRT you can occasionally work two reflexes within the same body system, such as the uterus and ovary or the neck and shoulder. The role of Zonal Triggers on the hands is discussed in detail in Chapter 3.

The uterus/prostate reflex has been selected here because it provides good practice in accessing the reflexes on the medial side of the hands and feet.

Method

1. Locate the uterus/prostate reflex on the medial (inside) palm side of your right hand with your left thumb and work it gently for a few seconds.

2. Place your weight-bearing right foot on a hard chair and locate the uterus/prostate foot reflex below the medial ankle bone and hold. Lean your leg well forwards on the chair for maximum weight-bearing pressure. Locate the Zonal Trigger pinprick sensation by using your left forefinger and begin pressing along the Zonal Trigger ankle-band while holding the dorsal reflex. A Zonal Trigger is usually, but not always, situated in the same zone as the reflex being worked. In this particular case it would be zone 1.

3. When a trigger point is not located anywhere in the band, return to the zone in which the reflex is situated and work a reflex in the centre of that zone.

4. Bring your left hand down to your right hand, which is working the foot, and locate with your left forefinger the uterus/prostate point on the medial side of the right hand at wrist level.

5. Place your right forefinger on the previously located Zonal Trigger. Your right thumb and forefinger are splayed apart as they touch the Zonal Trigger and uterus/prostate reflex.

6. Work all three points together. Hold for 30 seconds and then repeat on the left. Always conclude with the Pituitary Pinch and Harmoniser on both hands.

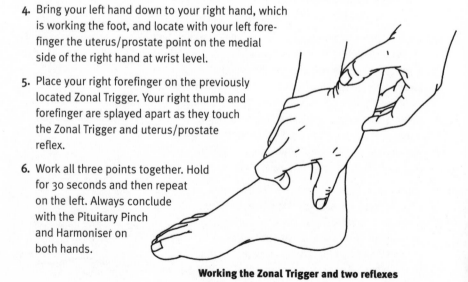

Working the Zonal Trigger and two reflexes

You could alternatively locate two reflexes on the hand and only one on the foot by locating the Zonal Trigger on the wrist of the hand. The foot, however, provides a more stable base for self-help work on the Zonal Triggers.

Self-help Diaphragm Rocking

Diaphragm Rocking is an extremely helpful aid to sleep, relaxation and even jet-lag. The key benefit of Diaphragm Rocking is that it appears to naturally prioritise and pump energy to the part of the body most in need. For full details see Chapter 3.

Self-help Diaphragm Rocking on the hands doesn't quite compare to the calming and relaxing sensation of someone gently rocking your hands or feet, but the actual results are just as effective.

This simple but profound technique can be applied as often as necessary, and is particularly helpful in combating insomnia. Diaphragm Rocking can be used on its own or to enhance one of the treatments described in this chapter.

Method

1. Hold your right hand upright in front of you, with your elbow to your side and palm facing you. Place your left thumb firmly on the solar plexus reflex of the palm near the metacarpal heads, situated between the first and second finger. Slightly lift your fingers up and over your thumb and bend them towards you.

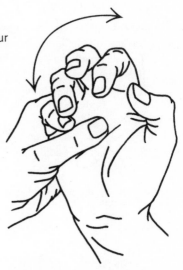

2. Hold your working thumb still near the hands of the metacarpal bones and let your hand do the work by gently rocking your fingers forwards and backwards in a rhythmic movement. Use your fingers to make at least 15 rocks per hand.

3. Repeat on the left hand.

Self-help Diaphragm Rocking

Lymphatic Stimulation

Lymphatic Stimulation and Diaphragm Rocking should ideally be introduced roughly halfway through a treatment, when the body has been treated with VRT and conventional reflexology.

Lymphatic stimulation can be used at any time or preferably before the Diaphragm Rocking technique described above – and can be applied for up to two minutes per hand. The body requires an efficient lymph system to remain healthy, and full details of this concept are to be found on page 69. This is a passive reflexology method that enhances VRT and conventional reflexology.

Method

This technique can also be applied to the dorsal (top) of weight-bearing hands and feet, which works equally well but is less relaxing. Each movement stimulates the abdominal organs, and the sweeping movements are designed to increase the flow of lymphatic fluid to help cleanse the body.

1. Place your right elbow on a cushion and hold your palm facing upwards and pointing back towards your body.

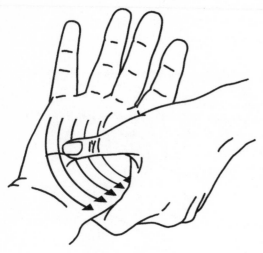

Lymphatic Stimulation

2. Place your left thumb on the palm of your right-hand diaphragm reflex below the middle finger, slightly towards the medial (inside) side of the hand, and in a sweeping movement make an arch with your thumb across all the abdominal reflexes, ending in the area of the lumbar spine. It is helpful to use a little cream here.

3. Repeat these movements five times so that the thumbs start a little further along the diaphragm reflexes of the hand and finish further down the lumbar spine nearer the heel of the hand. Ensure you press firmly on the bladder reflex on the fourth or fifth pass to stimulate the elimination of toxins and excess fluid from the body.

Self-help advanced techniques of the weight-bearing hands

Finger Pressure, Palmar Pressure, Knuckle Dusting and Palming are all useful techniques that can be applied to your own hands by using the methods for working on clients described in Chapter 4. These techniques are not essential but can greatly enhance a treatment.

Working the neural pathway reflexes on the hands

Working the neural pathways is an advanced technique that can be used from the second treatment onwards. The dorsal reflex, Zonal Trigger and corresponding neural pathway reflex are all found on the hand. The aim of this technique is to stimulate the working of the 31 pairs of cervical and spinal reflexes by connecting the appropriate corresponding organ reflex on the hand. See the illustration on page 60 for details.

Simultaneous self-help work on the hand neural pathways is restricted because you have only one working hand. The neural pathway reflex is worked first with your knuckle, and the other two reflexes are then treated separately. The only way you can simultaneously work the priority reflex, the neural pathway reflex and the Zonal Trigger is to work on your feet, which allows you to use both. Full details for all foot techniques are found in the companion book *Vertical Reflexology*.

To achieve the best results on the neural pathway reflexes it is important to use your knuckle or the medial (inside) edge of your thumb until you contact the priority reflex area using bone-on-bone. The cervical vertebrae reflexes start just below the medial thumbnail and the lumbar, sacral and coccyx reflexes are situated at the base of the wrist. You will feel a distinct pinprick sensation when you make contact with the correct neural pathway point. The lateral helper spine reflexes must be used when treating an actual spinal condition and, in this case, the corresponding Zonal Trigger is also found on the lateral side of the dorsal hand. The neural pathway reflex itself can then be located on the medial side of the hand and worked immediately.

Method

After applying basic self-help hand VRT you will have ascertained the main priority reflex that needs stimulating with the neural pathway reflex and the Zonal Trigger. The shoulder is used here as an example.

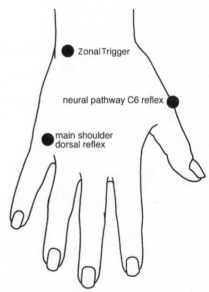

1. Briefly brush and press the reflexes around your wrists for a few seconds to activate the zones, then find the specific priority shoulder reflex on the dorsum (top) of the right hand and work it briefly.

2. Locate and work the Zonal Trigger simultaneously with the selected reflex point using your thumb and index finger.

3. Remove your finger and thumb, and with the knuckle of your working left hand or the side of the thumb, locate the appropriate neural pathway/spinal reflex. Work it firmly for 30

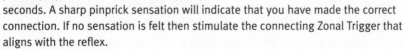

Self-help: the neural pathways

seconds. A sharp pinprick sensation will indicate that you have made the correct connection. If no sensation is felt then stimulate the connecting Zonal Trigger that aligns with the reflex.

4. Repeat on the other hand. If the problem is a right- or left-sided condition only then still treat the corresponding area of the three reflexes on your other hand to keep the zones in balance.

Self-help VRT nail-working

VRT nail-working is a very effective means of working the zones on your own nails from the passive or weight-bearing position of the hands. As with neural pathway reflexes, you will not be able to work three reflexes simultaneously but must work sequentially. It is helpful to press the pituitary reflex, nail-on-nail, on each hand before finding the dorsal hand reflex.

Nail-working on your passive hands

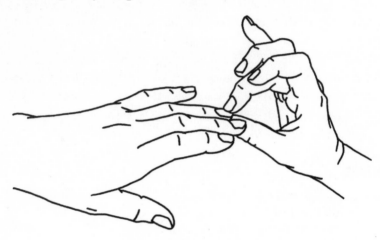

Working the five nail zones

Method

1. Take your left hand in your right hand and turn it so that it is facing palm down-wards. Place the four fingers of your right hand over the lateral (outside) edge of the top of your hand and put your index or third fingertip at wrist level on the top of the hand in zone 5, in alignment with the little finger.

2. Pinch down your hand in a line along the fifth metacarpal and continue down your finger in small bites until the tip of your index finger-pad touches the fingernail.

3. Arch your index finger and place the tip of its nail at the base of your little finger-nail. Edge your nail along the centre of the fingernail to the tip. It is essential that you lightly touch with nail-on-nail while firmly moving the pad of your forefinger along the pad of your finger until you reach the tip of your nail.

4. Return to the wrist and work zones 4 and 5 in this manner. Now turn your hand over and, using your left hand, hold your right hand and work your forefinger up from the wrist and then your thumb ending by working the nail in zones 1 and 2. Repeat on your left hand.

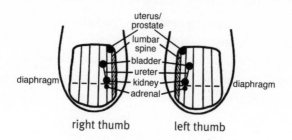

Nail reflexes for urinary conditions

Nail-working on your weight-bearing hands

The following instructions can be applied to the passive nails as well as the weight-bearing nails. The urinary system is used for this example. The spine, adrenal and uterus/prostate reflexes are also worked as they can act as helper reflexes when treating the urinary system.

Method

1. Press your right hand firmly on a flat surface. Locate the pituitary reflex in the middle of your thumbnail, nail-on-nail, and use it as an energiser/balancer to connect to urinary reflexes.

2. Briefly work around the wrists, Zonal Triggers and the spinal reflexes down the side of the thumb as described on pages 36–7 to make the body more receptive.

3. Again locate the pituitary reflex situated in the middle of your right thumbnail with your thumb-tip and hold for five seconds.

4. Now you can swiftly work each urinary and helper reflex in turn in the following sequence:

   - the adrenal, then briefly touch the pituitary reflex nail-on-nail for five seconds

   - the kidney and all other reflexes sequentially in the same manner:

     - the ureter

     - the bladder

     - the uterus/prostate

     - the lumbar spine

5. Repeat on the left hand.

6. Conclude with the self-help Harmoniser technique.

To complete, you can then introduce some fine-tuning advanced techniques such as Knuckle Dusting, Palmar Pressure, Finger Pressure and synergistic work.

VRT self-help treatments are essential maintenance

There is a misconception, even among reflexologists, that self-help reflexology is a rather sterile experience compared to an interactive treatment. VRT, on the other hand, allows the body to become much more receptive to our own touch, and the synergistic, neural pathway and nail-working methods enable us to obtain feedback and sensations from the reflexes as if we were being treated by a practitioner.

Key points to remember

- VRT self-help hand reflexology is a very accessible way of treating common ailments, administering first aid and general body maintenance.

- Teach your clients and friends these self-help techniques and they will be able to enhance your treatments between sessions.

- Always remember to place your weight-bearing hand on a firm, flat surface.

- Make sure you work in a comfortable position whether you are standing or sitting. Be aware of your posture and the positioning of your hands.

- Do not over-work the hands. Never stimulate any reflex for more than 30 seconds at a time when weight-bearing.

- Diaphragm Rocking can be used whenever desired for up to two minutes per hand.

- Use the Harmoniser in every treatment.

- Always start with your wrist reflexes and completely work one hand at a time.

- Drink water to help detoxify after treatments.

Part 2

Systems
of the body

Chapter 7

Hand VRT for specific ailments

Our bodies are usually amazingly resilient to the wear and tear of everyday life, not to mention emotional stresses. This is because the body has enormous adaptative mechanisms for coping with ill health, and it is often only when its resources are exhausted that we seek medical help or make a change in eating or other lifestyle habits. The delicate balance between good health and illness is very fragile and yet the miracle of life is that the body continues to repair, support and compensate for accidents, stress, poor diet and the general wear and tear of ageing.

The systems of the body comprise inter-related groups of organs, glands, nerves and skeletal structures that each work towards a specific function. In this section I briefly describe each system and provide advice on hand reflexology that can help heal common conditions. (See the guide to treating common ailments, page 169, for details of many other conditions.) I have also included information about other complementary therapies that can work with reflexology to bring about healing. For an overview of how these therapies work see page 180. Remember that reflexologists do not claim to cure or treat specific conditions; instead, they work with the appropriate systems of the body to stimulate the innate healing resources that lie within the body.

The systems of the body are:

- The neurological system. The entire body is controlled by the brain and the central nervous system. The spinal cord supplies nerves and relays messages to and from the brain to the appropriate parts of the body (Chapter 8).

- The skeletal system. This consists of the bones that protect and support the body (Chapter 9).

- The muscular system. There are three different types of muscle which support the skeletal system, give strength to the body and enable it to move (Chapter 10).

- The lymphatic system. This system deals with the disposal of waste in the body by means of lymph nodes, tissues and vessels (Chapter 11).

- The respiratory system. This system processes oxygen via the lungs to nourish the blood and discharge carbon dioxide (Chapter 12).

- The cardiovascular and circulatory system. This includes the heart and blood, which circulates through the veins, arteries and capillaries (Chapter 13).

- The digestive system. This processes food into chemical substances to nourish the body and excretes waste products (Chapter 14).

- The urinary system. This processes and eliminates toxins from the blood via the kidneys, which not only act as a filter for urine but also control the balance of many chemical functions in the body (Chapter 15).

- The endocrine system. This consists of ductless glands that produce hormones to stimulate and control many of the body's processes, including the metabolism (Chapter 16).

- The sense organs. These include the skin, ears, nose, tongue and eyes, all of which give the brain information about the body's environment (Chapter 17).

- The reproductive system. This consists of a series of functions to produce sperm, in the case of males, and eggs from the ovaries, in the case of females, to produce a baby (Chapter 18).

Options for applying techniques

Ideally, the specific treatments will form part of a 30- to 35-minute full hand reflexology treatment. For emergency help the specific techniques listed below can be used in isolation, as long as the basic VRT opening techniques on the wrists and spinal reflexes are introduced first. The treatments can also be used as self-help.

When treating a specific condition as part of a full hand reflexology treatment, use the following four applications:

- Basic hand VRT.

- Conventional hand reflexology including Body Brush, Diaphragm Rocking and Lymphatic Stimulation.

- To complete, fine-tune the weight-bearing hand reflexes with advanced VRT techniques including nail-working, with reference to the instructions listed below.

- Always conclude with the Harmoniser technique.

When you are treating a specific condition for first aid, or if time is limited:

- Brush quickly around the wrist reflexes on the weight-bearing hand to stimulate the Zonal Triggers.

- Work up and down the spinal reflexes on the medial (inside) side of the hand, from the edge of the thumb to the wrist. Work the other hand.

- To complete, apply the techniques suggested below for a specific condition.

To treat a specific condition with self-help hand VRT:

- Brush quickly around the wrist reflexes on the weight-bearing hand to stimulate the Zonal Triggers.

- Work up and down the spinal reflexes on the medial side of the hand, from the edge of the thumb to the wrist. Work the other hand.

- Use conventional self-help hand reflexology with Body Brush, Diaphragm Rocking and Lymphatic Stimulation (or skip this stage if you are giving yourself first-aid VRT).

- To complete: apply the techniques suggested in Chapters 8–18 for a specific condition.

Chapter 8

The neurological system

The neurological system consists of the central nervous system and the autonomic nervous system and includes the brain and the spinal cord. The central nervous system supplies information from the brain to the body and back via 12 pairs of cranial nerves at the base of the brain and 31 pairs of nerves that branch out down the length of the spinal cord to every part of the body. Working the neural pathways is an advanced VRT technique.

The information below is designed to give you a brief overview of how the central nervous system functions. You will not need to remember these nerves and their functions unless you are a professional reflexologist. Here your overall knowledge of how the body works, in conjunction with the chart of the central nervous system on page 60, will enable you to link the points of the neural pathway reflex with a part of the body that is imbalanced (see Chapter 4). The spinal nerves supply messages to every part of the body and if the spinal vertebrae protecting the spinal cord are compressed or damaged, then the corresponding organ can be affected also.

The cranial nerves

These stem from the base of the brain and supply functions within the head including the operation of the eyes, the sense of smell and the facial muscles.

The spinal nerves

These comprise:

- Eight pairs of cervical nerves – these emanate from the neck and include supply of functions to the lips, sinuses and throat.

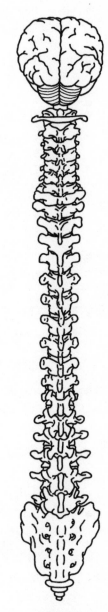

The brain and vertebrae protecting the spinal column

- Twelve pairs of thoracic nerves – these are situated in the upper thoracic spine and serve the lungs, adrenal glands and kidneys among others.

- Five pairs of lumbar nerves – these stem from the vertebrae of the lower back and are linked to parts of the body in the pelvic region and legs such as the reproductive organs, the bladder and the feet and ankles.

- Sacral and coccyx nerves – five sacral nerves serve the hips and buttocks, and the coccygeal nerve is linked to the rectum and anus.

The brain

- The brain stem – controls breathing, pulse and blood pressure.

- The cerebellum – regulates sleep, breathing, circulation and balance.

- The cerebrum (cerebral cortex) – comprises about 70 per cent of the brain and is divided into two hemispheres. It controls all the higher senses, communications and consciousness.

- The left hemisphere of the brain – is connected with our analytical thinking and also controls the right side of the body. It controls our speech and our writing and linguistic skills, as well as mathematical and logical application.

- The right hemisphere of the brain – is connected with our perceptions and non-verbal communication. It controls our spatial awareness, creativity and intuition.

- Some of the endocrine glands are situated above the cerebellum: the pituitary, pineal gland, hypothalamus and thalamus (see Chapter 16 for details).

The autonomic nervous system

The autonomic nervous system controls all the systems in the body over which we have no voluntary control. It has two parts – the sympathetic system and the parasympathetic system.

- The sympathetic nervous system has several functions, including increasing the heart rate, mobilising glucose and stimulating the sweat glands. It is involved in helping the body cope with increased activity.

- The parasympathetic nervous system helps to lower blood pressure and reduce the pace of the heartbeat, and is involved more with the functions of the body when at rest.

VRT and reflexology in general works on the autonomic nervous system in an indirect way by treating the whole body through the hands or feet and triggering a response where needed.

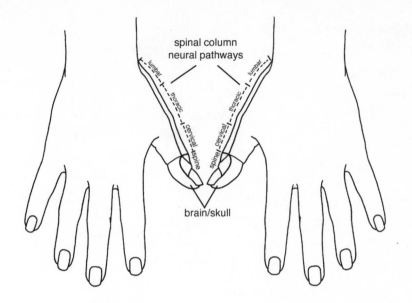

spinal column
neural pathways

lumbar

thoracic

cervical spine

spine cervical

thoracic

lumbar

brain/skull

Neurological reflexes on the hands

Insomnia

Insomnia is the inability to fall asleep or to remain asleep for an adequate amount of time. This complaint can take many different forms. Some people cannot get to sleep for hours; others fall immediately into a deep sleep for two or three hours and then lie awake for the rest of the night. Chronic insomnia over a long period of time can cause many health problems and places an enormous amount of stress on the sufferer. Symptoms can include poor concentration, chronic bouts of tiredness during the day, anxiety and stress, lack of coordination and headaches. Many parents with a crying baby, for example, feel that they can become almost zombie-like through lack of sleep. People need less sleep as they grow older but many of the elderly are constantly tired due to poor sleep patterns. Practical points to consider are:

- Make sure your bed is not too hard or too soft.
- Avoid eating large, rich meals late at night that may cause indigestion.
- Caffeine can cause wakefulness – avoid tea and coffee in the evenings.
- Ensure there is fresh air in your bedroom. Keep a window slightly open even if the central heating is on.
- Physical activity, such as a short walk before bed, may help.

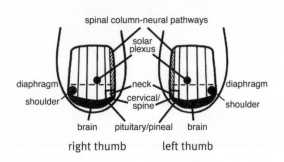

VRT techniques and priority reflexes

Condition Insomnia.

Main reflexes All toes, cervical spine, neck, shoulder, pituitary/pineal gland, solar plexus, brain.

Synergistic reflexes Solar plexus, pituitary/pineal.

Zonal Trigger Brain, use Diaphragm Rocking for two minutes per hand.

Nail reflexes for insomnia

VRT treatment

The key areas to help insomnia are the spinal reflexes, brain, cervical, spine, diaphragm and solar plexus reflexes.

- Use relaxation techniques and basic VRT, including tapping up and down the spinal reflexes for four to five passes per hand.
- Use the Spinal Twist (see page 14) to work the head, neck and thoracic reflexes thoroughly.
- Diaphragm Rocking is the key to helping insomnia and can be applied independently either to reflexology or VRT.
- Always work both hands when treating any condition as, for example, a left shoulder problem only treated on that side can cause referred pain in the right shoulder and neck area.
- Use the Whole Body Brush at least once.
- To end, work the diaphragm and solar plexus thoroughly.
- Include the two synergistic reflexes.
- Locate the neural pathway for the most affected area, such as tension in the neck or brain.
- Use Knuckle Dusting, concentrating on the fingers and thumbs.
- Work the five zones on each nail of the passive hands. Connect solar plexus and pituitary nail to dorsal reflexes.

Self-help VRT Use the Diaphragm Rocking techniques from Chapter 6. As you lie back work/rock each hand individually while simultaneously rocking both feet backwards and forwards in the same rhythm. Working the five zones on each nail of the passive hands is calming and soothing.

Optional complementary help

- **Aromatherapy** Lavender is a safe and gentle oil that helps induce sleep. A few drops can be used in the bath, or placed in an oil burner or on a hanky beside the pillow.

- **Herbal preparations** There are some very effective herbal remedies such as valerian, skullcap and hops, which can be taken as a tea or in tablet form. They can be purchased from chemists or health shops and often come in combination formulas, or you can see a qualified herbalist.

- **Homeopathy** Professional prescription is the suggested route but the following remedies achieve good results – Coffea, Nux Vomica, Ars. Alb. (all 6c or 30c potency).

- **Self-hypnosis and relaxation tapes** These are specially devised to help correct problematic sleeping patterns, and include positive affirmations and visualisations. A professional hypnotherapist can also help.

Chapter 9

The skeletal system

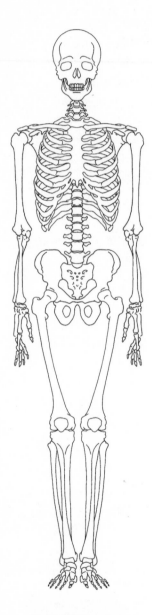

The skeletal system has two main functions: to protect vital organs and to allow movement. It is made up of 206 bones: 26 of them are in each foot and 27 are in each hand. The bones are dense tissue but are very much alive and active, and are made up of 45 per cent minerals, 30 per cent organic material and 25 per cent water. The bones undertake numerous chemical activities and produce and store minerals. The individual bones attach to the tendons and the muscles and assist in the formation of red blood cells and some white blood cells in the bone marrow.

The bones that protect the body are the skull which protects the brain, the ribcage which protects the heart and lungs, the spinal column which protects the spinal cord and the pelvic bones which offer some protection to abdominal organs.

The second function of the skeleton is to enable the body to move. It is an engineering marvel how a heavy body is supported and balanced by the feet and a thin pair of ankles. Likewise the skull and brain are extremely heavy and yet are comfortably supported on the narrow cervical vertebrae. The brain itself is about a fiftieth of our body weight.

Pressure on the organs can result if the spine is out of alignment; and a flexible, upright spine is the key to good health and vitality.

How VRT can help

VRT was discovered and developed after an elderly woman's hip freed up following a short application of reflexology on the weight-bearing feet. VRT has been particularly successful in loosening up the joints in the body and helping skeletal and mobility problems, and my catalogue of case histories from

The skeletal system

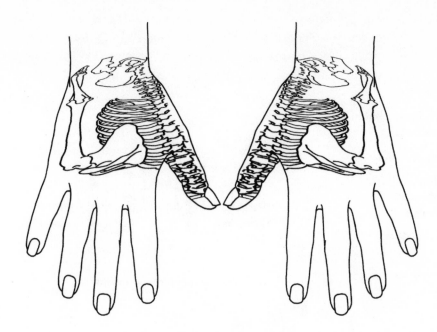

Skeletal reflexes on the hand

VRT practitioners contains more examples of improvement in mobility and lessening pain in this system than in any other system of the body. Synergistic VRT, where the hand and foot are worked simultaneously, appears to free up tight muscles and allows limbs to revert back to the correct position naturally. If you are new to VRT, I would advise you to treat and experiment with skeletal problems first, as they are very responsive to weight-bearing techniques.

Back problems

Shoulder, knee, hip and neck should be dealt with using the same techniques, but target specific reflexes as shown in the guide to treating common ailments on page 169.

Backache is a very general term that is liberally used to describe various conditions that stem from arthritis, trapped nerves, muscular spasm or displaced vertebrae to name but a few. Shoulder and neck problems can stem from a back injury and, conversely, they can cause backache by referred pain or because of an adverse change in posture. Many back problems originate from bad posture. This can cause a person to place more weight on one side of their body than on the other, resulting in problems as the body attempts to compensate.

Pain is a signal that there is a problem in that part of the body. By masking the pain, for example with painkillers, you treat the symptom, not the cause, and create a situation where you may strain the injury further. Over a period of time after an accident some people complain of tingling in a specific limb or limbs. This is a serious indication that nerves are damaged or trapped. Nerves take a very long time to heal and may not regenerate if the trapped nerve is not released.

VRT techniques and priority reflexes

Condition Back problems.

Main reflexes Full spine, hip/pelvic/sciatic, neck/shoulder.

Synergistic reflexes Pelvic/sciatic, neck/shoulder.

Zonal Trigger Appropriate spinal reflex.

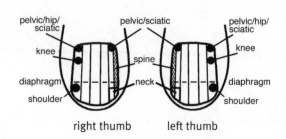

Nail reflexes for back problems

VRT treatment

The key areas to help ease a bad back are the spinal, neck and hip reflexes. Ensure you always work both hands when treating any condition, as a left shoulder problem can cause referred pain in the right shoulder and neck area, for example.

- Use relaxation techniques and basic VRT.
- Use Lymphatic Stimulation and Diaphragm Rocking.
- Use the Whole Body Brush at least once.
- Use the Spinal Twist.
- To end use full Fingertip Pressure.
- Apply Palmar Pressure – particularly work sciatic reflexes on the lateral side of the wrist.
- Include the two synergistic reflexes.
- Locate the neural pathway for the most affected area.
- Work specific nail reflexes. Connect key reflex with Zonal Trigger.
- Use Knuckle Dusting and Harmoniser.

Self-help VRT Repeat the above technique twice a day for all self-help VRT on the hands. Synergistic reflexology is an important extra method which can be used to increase the strength of the VRT when you work your hand and foot simultaneously.

Optional complementary help

- **Alexander Technique** You will have individual tuition over an extended period of time, as well as guidance in subtle methods of changing habits and attitudes, resulting in greater body awareness.

- **Massage** Remedial massage is often the best solution for injuries and chronic aches and pains.

- **Nutrition** Glucosamine sulphate appears to help arthritic conditions and is an extremely effective nutrient for the cartilage of joints, tendons and ligaments. As the cartilage begins to wear the body's natural ability to repair itself may be exceeded by the processes of cartilage erosion. Glucosamine sulphate contains a component called proteoglycan. This is a resilient structural material that acts as a cushion on the bone ends. Stabilised fish oil also works well in conjunction with this product, which is readily available in health shops and from nutritional supplement suppliers. It is worth noting that obesity can be a cause of some back pain. If this appears to be the case, sensible eating leading to controlled weight loss can ease the pressure on a weak back.

- **Osteopathy** It is advisable to have a series of appointments when dealing with a chronic long-term back problem, ensuring you give the body enough time to adjust and heal between treatments.

Chapter 10

The muscular system

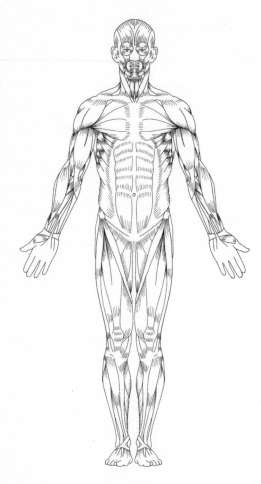

The muscular system

The muscular system is designed to allow movement and is responsible for about 50 per cent of our bodyweight. It is made up of two types of muscle – voluntary and involuntary.

Voluntary muscles

These are used for movement such as running or raising an arm, and are under our conscious control. They make up about 25 per cent of our body weight.

Gentle, regular exercise can tone up the muscles and enable them to retain their elasticity. At times muscles will go into spasm resulting in pain and decreased mobility. This can happen due to over- and under-usage, and the feeling of stiffness occurs because there are too many waste products in the system and the muscular fibres no longer slide over each other easily.

Involuntary muscles

These are not under direct conscious control – for example the heart and digestive system use muscles that are not consciously controlled by the brain. These muscles are called smooth muscles.

Tendons and Ligaments

Tendons are dense cords of connective tissue that connect the muscle to the bone. They have strength but no elasticity. When using conventional reflexology you need to work gently on the tendon but without applying pressure. However, this is not an issue when using VRT because the tendon is on the palm of the hand

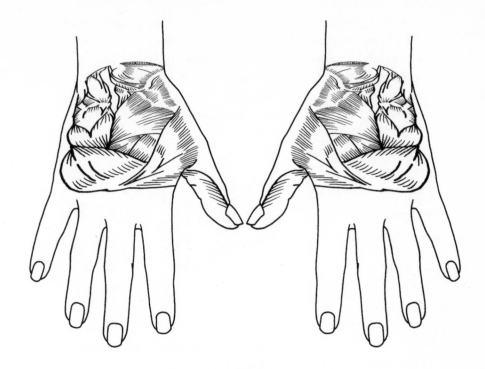

The muscular reflexes on the hands

and you will be working the dorsum (top). Ligaments have some elasticity and are connective tissues that hold bone to bone. Their slight elasticity prevents the bones from dislocating but still permits some freedom of movement.

Tendons and ligaments take longer to recover but VRT has shown remarkable results in freeing up tense muscles instantaneously. Shoulders and necks respond particularly well, as do hip joints. Many people who have had hip replacements have received relief from soreness and irritation of the surrounding muscles after VRT.

Sports injuries – muscular

Athletes, whether amateur or professional, run a high risk of injuring muscles and ligaments as well as bones and joints if they exercise vigorously or have an accident. Many sustain injuries after a break in activities or at the beginning of the season, when their bodies are not used to concentrated exertion. It is essential that anyone doing any form of sport or workouts in the gym should undertake a series of warm-up exercises first, so the muscles are stretched and warmed before being worked. Some injuries need no more attention than rest but others, such as a pulled calf muscle or hamstring, may need a complete break from exercise and help from a masseuse or physiotherapist to strengthen the muscles and increase the circulation of blood to the damaged tissues. It is important to be examined by a doctor or sports injury therapist after sustaining a painful or incapacitating injury, as there is a danger that short-term relief from ice-packs or pain-killing medication could mask the problem and the lack of pain would allow the person to put further strain on the injured part.

VRT techniques and priority reflexes

Condition Sports injuries.

Main reflexes Solar plexus, adrenals, hip/knee, hip/sciatic, spine, neck/shoulder, afflicted areas.

Synergistic reflexes Secondary afflicted area, spine.

Zonal Trigger Key afflicted area.

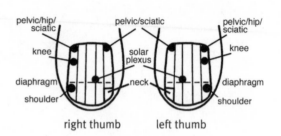

Muscular nail reflexes connected to sports injuries

VRT treatment

You will need to start with several minutes of relaxation techniques and basic VRT, as well as concentrated work on the spine (Spinal Twist) and pelvic area.

- Use Lymphatic Stimulation and Diaphragm Rocking.
- To end use Palmar Pressure.
- Locate the neural pathway for the key referral area and connect with Zonal Trigger.
- Use Knuckle Dusting.
- Use Palming – if appropriate reflexes can be reached.
- Work the Endocrine Flush (see Chapter 5) and concentrate on the adrenal gland.
- Nail-work on secondary and key referral areas.
- Use the Harmoniser to finish.
- Show the client three priority reflexes to work on the weight-bearing hand twice daily between treatments.

Self-help VRT The above techniques can be applied in the self-help mode. It is also important to apply synergistic reflexology on the hands and feet to the three priority reflexes. Work the reflexes vigorously and then use the Harmoniser.

Optional complementary help

- **Aromatherapy** An aromatherapist will massage the body, paying special attention to the affected area, and will apply a base or carrier oil mixed with drops of specific essential oils such as lavender to help with pain, or black pepper, ginger or marjoram to improve circulation.

- **Homeopathy** A homeopath will prescribe a very specific remedy based on a detailed consultation. For example, Ruta or Rhus Tox in potency 6, with one pill taken three times daily, is often helpful in the treatment of sprains and strains of the muscles and ligaments.

- **Massage** A masseuse will use deep tissue massage to help cure tensions in the muscles and stiffness in the joints as well as aiding in general relaxation of the body.

- **Osteopathy** An osteopath will treat the whole person with manipulative therapy on the framework of the bones, joints, muscles and specific ligaments.

Chapter 11

The lymphatic system

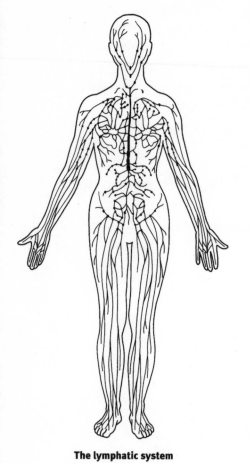

The lymphatic system

The lymphatic system comprises lymph vessels and lymph nodes. The lymph system is absolutely crucial to the health of the body as its role is to carry waste matter, excess fluid and toxins from the body's cells and tissues. The white blood cells in the body are known as lymphocytes and it is essential for the body to maintain the correct white blood cell count in its fight against disease. The tonsils, adenoids, spleen and thymus gland are also part of the lymphatic system.

There are two main drainage points in the body for lymph: the thoracic duct and the right lymphatic duct. The thoracic duct drains waste products from the legs, the pelvic and abdominal area and the left half of the upper body including the head. The right lymphatic duct lies at the base of the neck and drains fluid from the right side of the torso and head.

One of the roles of the lymphatic system is to remove large proteins from the body tissue and return them into the circulatory system for excretion. There are about 100 lymph nodes situated all over the body and many are found in the neck area. They can be as large as a peanut and as small as a pinhead. They act as lymph filters to prevent infection passing into the bloodstream. The classic case of painful swollen glands is the result of the lymph nodes being overwhelmed by toxins due to illness or infection in the body; they swell as they cannot process the waste products quickly enough.

The lymph system also has a vital role to play in supporting the immune system, and a healthy lymph system means a healthy body as disease and bacteria are efficiently eliminated.

Tissue fluid

This is colourless and is derived from blood plasma. Tissue fluid seeps through the capillaries and, unlike blood, it is not pumped from the heart but is moved by exercise and deep intakes of air into the lungs. When the tissue fluid reaches the lymph vessels it is called lymph.

The tonsils and adenoids

These are part of the lymph system and are situated at the back of the nasal cavity.

The spleen

This is a major filter system for damaged cells which also stores iron and breaks down old red blood cells. The spleen itself is comprised of lymphoid tissue.

The thymus

This is a gland that plays an important role in the immune system of children and shrinks as adulthood is reached. Its function is hormonal and it stimulates the body to produce lymphocytes and lymph tissue. The role of the thymus in adults is being reviewed as there is a suggestion that it is actively involved in the

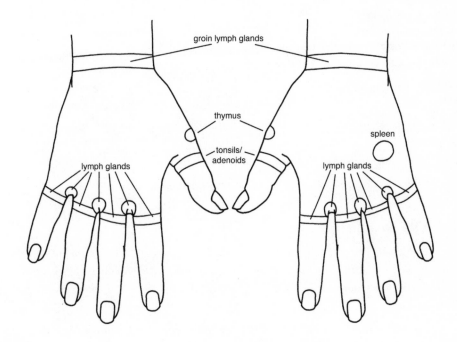

The lymphatic reflexes on the hand

production of T-lymphocytes, which are vital in the body's fight against tumour-producing cells.

Reflexology has always achieved impressive results when it comes to lymph drainage and related conditions such as oedema in the feet. With VRT lymph drainage is even more effective, as the standing position can accelerate the progress of fluid through the body. This results in a reduction of fluid, and a healthier lymphatic system can be noticed immediately. Often the improvements in lymph drainage are more permanent or only require a monthly VRT treatment to keep the problem at bay. In many people with oedema, the feet are too swollen to be worked, so the possibility of working on the weight-bearing hands is invaluable.

Oedema

Oedema means water retention and swollen feet, legs and ankles can occur when the circulation is slow or when water leaks from the blood and accumulates in the tissues. Water retention is common in pregnant and premenstrual women. Severe problems can arise with water retention due to kidney and heart conditions. Putting the feet up on a stool helps and many sufferers wear elasticated stockings when travelling by air to counteract the swelling and prevent deep vein thrombosis.

VRT techniques and priority reflexes

Condition Oedema.

Main reflexes Kidneys, adrenals, bladder, solar plexus/diaphragm, heart, lymph/neck, chest, lymph/groin, afflicted area.

Synergistic reflexes Kidney, lymph/groin.

Zonal Trigger Work key afflicted area.

Diaphragm Rocking Two to three minutes.

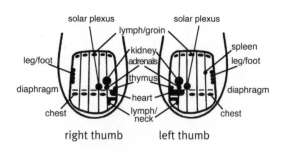

Nail reflexes for oedema

VRT treatment

Use relaxation techniques and basic VRT, working the lymphatic area three times as well as the groin reflexes. If the feet are painful and swollen always work the hands. For synergistic reflexology, just brush the reflexes or lightly press the feet or legs.

- Use Lymphatic Stimulation for at least one minute per hand, as well as Diaphragm Rocking.

- To end, locate the neural pathway – afflicted area or lymphatics.
- Use Knuckle Dusting.
- Use Palming several times over lymphatic and afflicted areas if possible.
- Nail-work on thumbs and preferably all nails – connect with the Zonal Trigger for the afflicted area of lymphatics (usually groin reflexes).
- Use the Harmoniser to finish.

Self-help VRT As above, but pay special attention to any particular area of swelling on the feet, and work the corresponding part of the hands and wrists. For abdominal bloating, use Lymphatic Stimulation for two to three minutes, and finish by working the afflicted area reflex with the connecting techniques for the nails (see Chapter 5).

Optional complementary help

- **Aromatherapy** This therapy can help the circulation and reduce the swelling in the limbs.
- **Herbal Medicine** A medical herbalist will prescribe a natural diuretic such as a dandelion infusion.
- **Nutrition** You will be advised to cut out salt, and your general health and diet will be scrutinised.

Chapter 12

The respiratory system

Breath is life. Most adults breathe over 13,000 litres of air a day and although the body can survive for days without water and weeks without food, we would be dead in a few minutes without air. Every minute we breathe in and out about 15 times. The respiratory system organs take in oxygen and exhale carbon dioxide and some water. The purpose of breathing is to oxygenate the blood upon which every cell depends. The system is divided into the upper and lower respiratory tract. As a person inhales this is called inspiration and as the air is expelled from the mouth and nose this is called expiration.

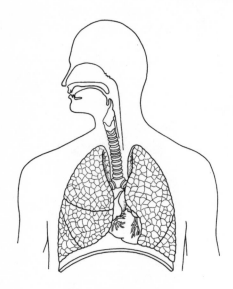

The respiratory system

Upper respiratory tract organs

These include the mouth, throat, larynx, cilia (filters) and sinus cavities in the head. As air passes through the nose it is filtered and warmed before passing into the lungs.

Lower respiratory tract organs

These include the windpipe (trachea), the bronchi and the lungs. The lungs comprise the alveoli (air sacks), bronchioles and bronchial tubes.

The lungs are the main organs of the respiratory tract and the diaphragm is a large, muscular wall that points upwards towards the lungs. When it contracts, during inspiration, the atmospheric pressure on the lungs decreases, causing the air to rush in. When the opposite happens and the diaphragm relaxes air rushes out. The air breathed in contains the oxygen that passes into the millions of alveoli in the lungs. In turn the alveoli pass oxygen into the capillaries and on into the bloodstream. At the same time carbon dioxide is extracted from the blood, and is then expelled through the mouth and nose.

We owe it to ourselves to breath more deeply, giving ourselves plenty of fresh air, and to protect our lungs from the damage of cigarette smoke and chemical pollution. Reflexologists can often tell if a person smokes, or has smoked, because the lung reflexes have a granular feel.

Asthma and bronchitis respond well to VRT as the top of the hand or foot can be worked vigorously to help desensitise or decongest the lungs. Asthmatics can also be taught to control their breathing patterns, in much the same way as professional singers benefit from using breathing techniques.

Working the breath for calm and energy

Breathing is something we literally do from the moment we are born until that last breath leaves us. Plainly all of us breathe and unless we have a medical problem, we are not usually conscious of it, but some ways of breathing are better for health, energy, confidence and voice than others.

The shallow upper chest pattern of breathing that becomes the habitual pattern for many of us encourages excess tension in the muscles of the upper chest, shoulders, neck and throat. Taking more frequent, shallow breaths can give our bodies a sense of pressure, which can even turn to panic if we are under stress. Then the blood pressure rises, the heart beats faster, there may be an adrenalin surge and we feel more anxious.

Lower breathing – also called central breathing, or inter-costal diaphragmatic breathing – is the method taught in yoga, Pilates, relaxation, martial arts and most physical training. The lower part of the chest should expand as the breath enters and contract as the breath leaves. The lungs behave a bit like balloons – when air enters a balloon, it expands – when air leaves, the sides of the balloon move in.

Working the breath

- Sit or lie comfortably with your back and head supported.

- Put one hand lightly just above your waistband and one just below. Feel the warmth or pressure of your hands and see if you can focus the breath to rise and fall there for a minute or two and just observe that breath entering and leaving your body.

- Pull the abdominal muscles in and out a few times. Now, as you pull in on those muscles, breathe out whilst making a long 'shhhhh' sound. Do this several times in quick succession. As you are doing it, notice that you do not have to take a breath in as the breath just drops in – low and centred as it should be. You can gradually build up to 25 per cent more lower breathing muscle involvement – all without strain.

If you are a habitual upper chest breather, this will probably feel most self-conscious and unnatural – but if practised daily for two weeks or so, it will gradually centre and settle until it feels more normal.

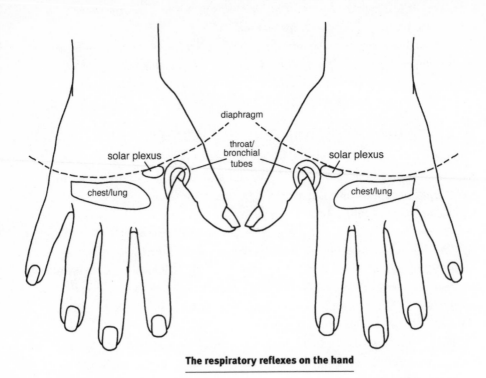

The respiratory reflexes on the hand

Bronchial problems

Bronchial problems usually result in a wet or dry cough. A dry cough is caused by inflammation or infection in the bronchial tubes. A cough with phlegm is often caused by a cold, which leaves mucous on the lungs. Chronic coughs can be due to allergy, heavy smoking or asthma. A persistent cough can indicate a serious problem, so always see a doctor.

VRT techniques and priority reflexes

Condition Bronchial problems.

Main reflexes Chest/lung, throat, lymphatics, thoracic.

Synergistic reflexes Throat, chest/lung.

Zonal Trigger Lymphatics.

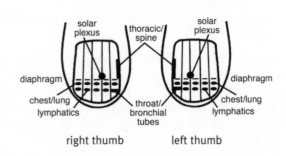

Nail reflexes for the bronchial problems

VRT Treatment

- Use relaxation techniques and Basic VRT, working the chest/lung lymphatic area.
- Use Lymphatic Stimulation and Diaphragm Rocking.
- To end use Plantar Pressure.
- Locate the neural pathway – upper thoracic reflex or lymphatics.
- Use Knuckle Dusting.
- Use Palming several times over the chest area.
- Nail-work on the thumbs for chest/lung – connect with Zonal Trigger.
- Use the Harmoniser to finish.

Self-help VRT Work the chest/lung/lymphatic and sinus reflexes for a few minutes several times a day, especially the webbing of the hand. Work the weight-bearing hand reflexes at least twice in the morning and evening.

Optional complementary help

- **Aromatherapy** Use sandalwood for dry coughs. Frankincense, tea tree, eucalyptus, thyme or lavender oils can be inhaled with steam or mixed with a carrier oil and rubbed into the throat or neck.
- **Herbal Medicine** Health food shops stock excellent herbal preparations for dry or productive coughs or see a herbalist.
- **Homeopathy** Bryonia is a familiar remedy for coughs but accurate prescribing is needed to target the precise type of cough for maximum benefit.
- **Nutrition** A nutritionist may advise taking at least 1000 mg of Vitamin C per day, echinacea to boost the immune system or garlic capsules to help clear the sinuses. Elderberry juice, fresh or a proprietary brand, is excellent as a flu/bronchial virus inhibitor.
- **Osteopathy** Soft-tissue manipulation can help to shift mucous and ease tension in the back and ribs caused by coughing.
- **Phytobiophysics** This therapy can offer constitutional help for persistent coughs, especially if tension or stress is a possible cause.

Chapter 13

The cardiovascular and circulatory system

The heart

The heart is a muscle that is central to the cardiovascular and circulatory system and is vital for life. Its role is to pump oxygen and the nutrients the body requires to every cell and tissue in the body via the blood, which flows through the arteries, veins and capillaries. The circulating blood also removes waste products and carbon dioxide. The heart is positioned on the left side of the body in the thoracic cavity, is about the size of a small fist, and weighs about 255 g. In a 24-hour period the heart will have pumped about 36,000 litres of blood around the body.

The heart has four chambers – the right and left atria (upper) and the right and left ventricles (lower). Blood vessels leading from the heart are called arteries, and they carry blood to all parts of the body. The aorta is the largest artery.

The blood

Blood has four main components: plasma, erythrocytes (red corpuscles), leukocytes (white corpuscles) and platelets. The pulmonary artery carries the blood from the heart to the lungs, where it discharges the carbon dioxide and picks up the oxygen to be carried through the bloodstream.

The freshly oxygenated blood carries nutrients throughout the body to the cells by means of arteries and capillaries. The veins despatch carbon dioxide back to the heart and lungs to be discharged.

One of the key factors in reflexology is that it improves circulation and in doing so increases the vitality of the body. The circulatory system is

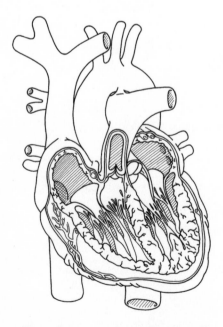

The cardiovascular and circulatory system

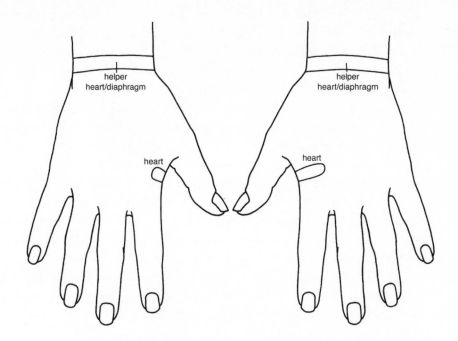

helper
heart/diaphragm

helper
heart/diaphragm

heart

heart

The cardiovascular reflexes on the hand

the front line for maintaining the body's immunity. The cardiovascular system sends out antibodies to fight potential disease all the time, and it is essential that the antibodies are directed to vulnerable areas in the body. A sluggish circulatory system means this does not happen as effectively. With VRT the heart reflexes, and the entire dorsal area, should be worked thoroughly to stimulate the circulation and increase immunity to disease. VRT heart helper reflexes on the wrists and ankles help to balance the entire cardiovascular system.

Angina and stroke

Angina occurs when the demand for blood exceeds the supply of the coronary arteries. This is usually due to coronary artery atheroma, or narrowing of the arteries. The result is severe chest pain in the centre of the chest.

A stroke is a sudden attack of weakness that affects one side of the body and results in an interruption of the flow of blood to the brain due to thrombosis, haemorrhage or embolus. It can result in severe paralysis and death or can be a mild passing weakness.

Never try to diagnose a heart condition and never change or discontinue any medical care or medication. The following gentle, non-invasive VRT hand techniques are used to complement a patient's medical treatment, aiming to support the body and bring about better circulation and balance so that the heart is better able to cope under stress. If there is ever any negative change in a person's medical condition that causes concern, call a doctor immediately. VRT has appeared to be instrumental in accelerating the return of some faculties after a stroke, and many angina sufferers discover they can limit the number of attacks if self-help VRT is regularly applied to the hands.

These same general techniques are helpful in regulating high blood pressure (hypertension) or low blood pressure (hypotension). Blood pressure falls when a person is resting and rises when the body is stressed, physically exerted or alerted to danger. In hypertension blood pressure remains high even when the person is at rest. The causes of hypertension include a build-up of cholesterol in the blood, hardening of the arteries and stress, as well as smoking and excessive alcohol. If you are treating someone who is on medication for high blood pressure, advise them to have their blood pressure checked regularly as they may need less medication if their blood pressure begins to lower naturally.

Hypotension is rarely dangerous when it is chronic. However, problems can arise when blood pressure suddenly drops and the arteries do not constrict quickly enough to maintain a sufficient supply of blood to the brain. This can result in dizziness or fainting.

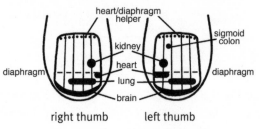

Nail reflexes for heart conditions

VRT techniques and priority reflexes

Condition Angina and stroke.

Main reflexes Heart helper reflexes, heart, lung, diaphragm, sigmoid colon, thoracic arm, toes, helper heart on wrist, spine, brain, kidneys, affected areas.

Synergistic reflexes i. Angina: sigmoid colon, diaphragm. ii. Stroke: wrist reflex and affected area.

Zonal Trigger i. Heart. ii. Brain: alternative side to paralysis.

Diaphragm Rocking Two minutes.

VRT techniques and priority reflexes

Condition High and low blood pressure (hypertension and hypotension).

Main reflexes Kidneys, diaphragm, solar plexus, all glands, thyroid, heart and helper heart on wrist.

Synergistic reflexes Heart and kidneys.

Zonal Trigger Diaphragm.

Diaphragm Rocking Two to three minutes.

VRT treatment

Start with relaxation techniques and basic VRT – work the fingers three times, work the thoracic calf four times on each arm, and tap on the spinal reflexes vigorously.

- Use Lymphatic Stimulation/Diaphragm Rocking and Spinal Twist.
- To end use full Fingertip Pressure.
- Locate the neural pathway for the most affected area; heart helper or brain should be left for second treatment, as neural pathway work is usually too powerful on a first treatment.
- Use Knuckle Dusting.
- Whole Body Brush.
- Use Palming.
- Nail-working – work the heart reflex on the thumbnail and secondary nail for angina and the brain reflex on the thumb and secondary nails for stroke.
- Use the Harmoniser to finish.

Self-help VRT As above for angina, blood-pressure problems and strokes. Work the spine and all brain reflexes on a daily basis. If an arm or leg is affected work up and down weight-bearing zone 5 several times a day and pinch the five zones on the little fingernail nail-on-nail.

To help to prevent an angina attack: sit down and place the weight-bearing hand on a low flat table beside you; brush your thumb across the left wrist helper heart reflex. Drink a glass of tepid water to help to rehydrate the heart. This should never take the place of aerosol or under tongue medication if it is required.

Optional complementary help

- **Aromatherapy** A gentle massage with oils such as lavender, rose or sandalwood can help release tension if blood pressure is high.
- **Breathing techniques** Learn the basic calming breaths as described in Chapter 12.
- **Hypnotherapy** There are tapes available to help overcome tension.
- **Massage** This therapy can help to relieve tension and improve the circulation and movement to an affected limb.
- **Nutrition** A low-fat balanced diet with plenty of fresh fruits, vegetables and exercise is one of the key factors in the prevention of heart disease. Vitamin E and Omega 3 stabilised fish oils are often prescribed by nutritionists.
- **Psychotherapy and counselling** Many stroke victims are traumatised by their sudden decline and need help to come to turns with it.

Chapter 14

The digestive system

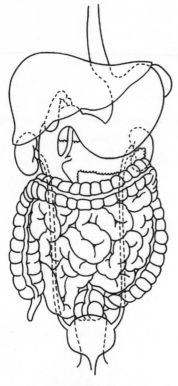

The digestive system

The digestive system begins at the mouth, where the food is chewed by 32 teeth with the help of saliva and the tongue. The pharynx passes the food to the stomach via the oesophagus and from there it travels to the small intestine – which is made up of the duodenum, jejunum and ileum – where most of the digestive processes take place. The liver, gall bladder and pancreas also aid digestion. The waste matter passes into the large intestine (bowel) via the ileocecal valve that permits outflow of the intestinal contents, which are expelled from the rectum.

The colon is divided into sections as it curves its way around the abdomen: the ascending colon passes up on the right side of the abdomen and turns left at the hepatic flexure to become the transverse colon. It then turns down at the splenic flexure to become the descending colon. The sharp bend near the end of the colon is called the sigmoid flexure, which then becomes the rectum leading on to the anus at the point of exit from the body.

The digestive system converts food into substances that the body is able to absorb and use. The body needs a variety of foods to supply it with the vital materials for energy and heat. The essential chemicals in food are absorbed and processed to help the growth and repair of the body that are essential to life.

How VRT can help

VRT and reflexology work towards normalising bodily functions, and the same reflexes are worked whether the bowels are too active or too inactive. VRT and synergistic reflexology are extremely successful in treating Irritable Bowel Syndrome (IBS), but lasting success is only achieved when dietary habits are addressed at the same time.

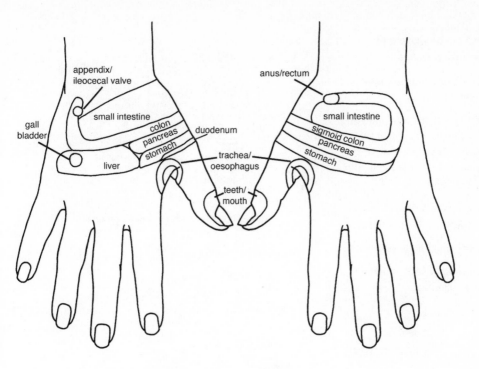

appendix/
ileocecal valve

anus/rectum

gall
bladder

small intestine

small intestine

colon

sigmoid colon

pancreas

pancreas

duodenum

stomach

stomach

trachea/
oesophagus

liver

teeth/
mouth

Digestive reflexes on the hands

Irritable Bowel Syndrome

Irritable Bowel Syndrome sufferers can experience alternating bouts of diarrhoea and constipation, plus abdominal pain and distension caused by a build-up of gas. Anxiety and tension can accompany this often embarrassing condition, as can mucous in the faeces, nausea and loss of appetite.

'We are what we eat' is an old and familiar adage, but the truth is that we are what we absorb. If we have a congested and lethargic colon we are unable to digest the nutrients we eat. A nutritionist can prescribe a variety of supplements and give dietary advice, which may help. Allergy testing can also highlight foods to which a person has become intolerant. Many headaches reflect a malfunction in another part of the body rather than in the head itself – in fact some clients presenting with headaches suffer from bowel disorders and these disappear once the digestive system has been treated. Naturopaths will often insist on first treating the digestive system, particularly the bowel, before concentrating on other ailments in the body. They believe that if the body's waste-disposal system is faulty, other organs or glands will not respond because the entire body will be toxic and compromised.

VRT techniques and priority reflexes

Condition Irritable Bowel Syndrome.

Main reflexes Large and small intestines, ileocecal valve, solar plexus, diaphragm, adrenals, cervical and lumbar spine, liver.

Synergistic reflexes Cervical and lumbar spine, adrenals.

Zonal Triggers Large intestine.

Diaphragm Rocking Two to three minutes.

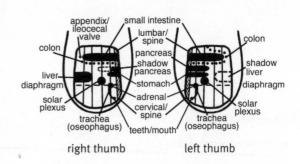

right thumb   left thumb

Nail reflexes for Irritable Bowel Syndrome

VRT treatment

- Use several minutes of relaxation techniques and basic VRT, as well as concentrated work on the cervical and lumbar spine (plus Spinal Twist) and abdominal area.

- Use Lymphatic Stimulation for one minute per hand and Diaphragm Rocking.

- To end locate the neural pathway – the most tender point on the large intestine – and connect with Zonal Trigger.

- Use Palming – concentrate on the small and large intestine. Work across the transverse colon reflex.

- Work the nail-pituitary reflex simultaneously with the adrenal gland to relieve tension. Repeat on the other hand.

- Work the two synergistic reflexes.

- Nail-work on the secondary and intestinal reflexes connected with the most tender reflex.

- Use the Harmoniser to finish.

- Show the client three priority reflexes to work on the weight-bearing hand twice daily between treatments, or when there is discomfort.

Self-help VRT As above, but also pinch down the spinal reflexes using Fingertip Pressure. Work the whole grid system on each of the thumbnails, nail-on-nail, and work the hand itself with your knuckle on either the T12 or the L1 neural pathway reflex. Work the digestive reflexes on your palm or weight-bearing hand, as well as the Lymphatic Stimulation techniques, whenever you experience abdominal discomfort.

Optional complementary help

- **Applied Kinesiology** A kinesiologist uses muscle testing as a means of determining what foods should be eliminated or added to the diet. They can also prescribe supplements and check on the body's muscle response to determine the root cause of the problem.

- **Bach Flower Remedies** Specific remedies such as Aspen and Mimulus are helpful when anxiety precipitates digestive problems or when the distressing IBS symptoms provoke fear and tension.

- **Homeopathy** Two helpful remedies are Nux Vomica and Lycopodium.

- **Nutritionist or naturopath** Seeing a qualified therapist is often the best way forwards if food intolerances are causing digestive problems and headaches.

- **Remedial massage** Deep tissue massage is excellent for relaxation, curing tensions and physical problems. As many bowel problems are stress related, this can be an excellent complementary therapy.

- **Self-hypnosis and relaxation tapes** These are specially devised to help people to cope with many physical and emotional problems, and include positive affirmations and visualisations. Professional help may also be beneficial.

Chapter 15

The urinary system

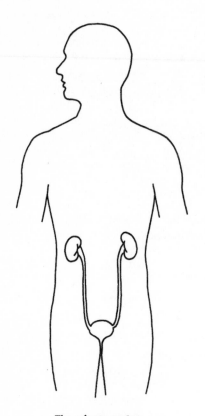

The urinary system

The urinary system comprises the two kidneys, the ureters that transport urine to the bladder, and the urethra which in turn passes the urine out of the body. The bladder and kidneys are well protected – the bladder by the pelvic and hip bones, and the kidneys by the ribcage – so neither are particularly susceptible to injury or knocks. The urinary tract is a much more vulnerable part of the system, and can be prone to infections and inflammation, as stale urine can accumulate and breed bacteria. Sterile urine contains no microbes, but infection and bacteria are easily transmitted to the urinary system via the urethra. Women are particularly susceptible because the female urethra is only 4 cm in length and external bacteria are easily transmitted, causing inflammation of the bladder (cystitis) and urgent need for urination.

Men often suffer from frequency of urination and other urinary problems in later life, and this is usually caused by an enlarged prostate gland. Several random surveys conducted by the popular press have discovered that the majority of men do not know what the prostate gland is or where it is situated! This indicates that only a very small proportion of males check their prostate regularly to detect any change in size or tenderness which could indicate benign enlargement or possibly the slow-growing but potentially fatal prostate cancer. It is usually a negative change in urinary function that alerts doctors to a potential health problem in this area.

The kidneys

The kidneys are bean-shaped and are each about 10 cm long, 5 cm wide, and 2.5 cm deep. They are situated at the back of the body in the area of the waistline; the right kidney is positioned slightly lower than the left one. The kidney is the

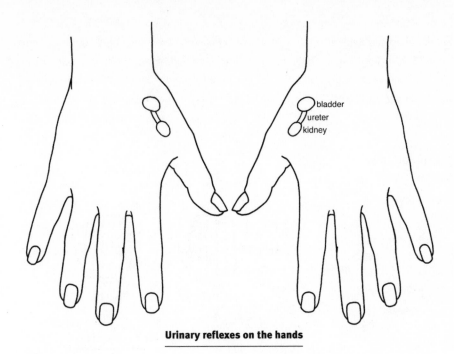

bladder
ureter
kidney

Urinary reflexes on the hands

master chemist of the body and its function is to separate waste products from the blood and to keep it chemically balanced despite the variations in foods and liquids consumed. Much of the water, salts, glucose and some urea are processed through the kidneys and returned to the bloodstream, but the waste and excess becomes urine. Up to 180 litres of fluid are processed daily by the kidneys, and 1.5 litres is excreted by the body as urine.

The ureters and urethra

These are thin, muscular tubes, up to 30 cm long, that carry urine from the kidneys to the bladder, which is a very elastic, muscular bag or sac that has a capacity to hold 600 ml or more of urine. There is an urge to urinate when the bladder is full and the urine is consciously released via the urethra, which is a narrow, muscular tube only 4 cm long in a woman and 20 cm long in a man.

Bladder problems – frequency of urination

Reflexologists work all the reflexes of the urinary system to help it function efficiently and VRT has proved extremely helpful in helping cystitis, bladder infections, pressure from an enlarged prostate gland or a weakened pelvic floor after childbirth resulting in stress incontinence. Several reports have been received of kidney stones being passed naturally after receiving VRT or reflexology. The kidney reflexes on the dorsum (top) of the hand and the plantar (soles) of the feet can often feel tender but can be worked vigorously to stimulate the function of the entire urinary system. Some of the newer hand and heel weight-bearing VRT techniques have been used to help stimulate the bladder reflexes. Clients have occasionally reported that they feel their bladder capacity has increased since receiving VRT, and that their sphincter control has improved. In many cases bladder problems are curable and treatable once accurately diagnosed by a doctor.

VRT techniques and priority reflexes

Condition Frequency of urination.

Main reflexes Bladder, kidneys, ureters, lumbar spine, adrenals, prostate (in men, if enlarged).

Synergistic reflexes Lumbar spine, ureters, prostate (if indicated).

Zonal Trigger Bladder.

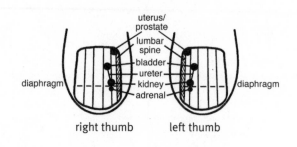

Nail reflexes for bladder problems

VRT treatment

Start with relaxation techniques, basic VRT, and vigorous working and tapping on the lumbar spinal reflexes, as well as the Spinal Twist.

- Use Lymphatic Stimulation/Diaphragm Rocking/Whole Body Brush.
- To end use Palmar Pressure.
- Work the neural pathway for the bladder on second treatment.
- Use Knuckle Dusting.
- Nail-working – work the bladder and lumbar spine reflexes (and the prostate reflex when required) on the thumbs and secondary nails for kidneys, ureters and adrenals. Apply the Urinary Flush (see Chapter 5) – work both hands at once.
- Use the Harmoniser to finish.

Self-help VRT As above: work the bladder reflex on the weight-bearing hand several times a day and work into the ureter and kidney reflexes on the palm with your thumb or knuckles. Work the prostate reflex if required, especially if urine retention is a problem.

Optional complementary help

- **Applied Kinesiology** The bladder and kidney meridians can be strengthened through these techniques.

- **Herbal medicine** Products containing saw palmetto may be prescribed for prostate problems and specific herbal formulas can be prescribed for cystitis.

- **Nutrition** Cranberry capsules or juice are often prescribed to help prevent bacteria building up in the bladder. Dietary advice is to limit alcohol, caffeine, artificial colourants and sweeteners, as all are known to irritate the bladder.

- **Homeopathy** Preparations such as Cantharis are prescribed to combat urinary frequency.

- **Psychotherapy** Frequency of urination can sometimes be emotionally based and, if no physical cause can be found, it can be worth exploring the emotional factors, especially if anxiety is present.

Chapter 16

The endocrine system

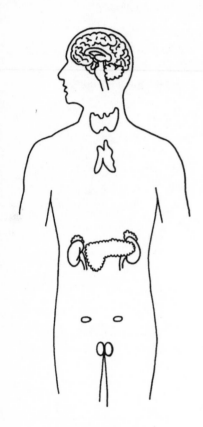

The endocrine system

The endocrine system is the hormonal system which regulates the body's many metabolic processes and is essential for regulating its chemical functions. Endocrine gland secretions work to control changes in the body, including the growth rate and sexual functions. They are ductless glands that secrete hormones into the bloodstream – they are carried around until they reach the part of the body targeted to respond to a particular hormone. These glands function independently but depend on a general hormonal balance in the body to operate properly.

The pituitary gland

This gland is often referred to as the master gland, as its role is to regulate the other endocrine glands. The pituitary gland is the size of a pea and is situated on a stalk at the base of the brain. It works closely with the hypothalamus.

The hypothalamus

The hypothalamus has many functions, including influencing our sexual behaviour. It also has centres that determine whether something is painful or pleasant. It is responsible for controlling body temperature, appetite, satiety and thirst, and regulating the heart, and it controls the amount of hormones secreted by the pituitary gland.

The pineal gland

This is a minute gland in the third ventricle of the brain which influences behaviour and mood swings and secretes melatonin, which is believed to be a light receptor. The correct amount of melatonin is essential for our body-clock to work properly.

The thymus gland

This gland is part of the lymphatic system (see Chapter 11) but is also an endocrine gland. It contains lymphocytes that help the body defend itself against disease. It is located in the upper part of the chest and remains active until puberty, at which point it begins to shrink (although it may have some adult function).

The thyroid and parathyroid glands

These glands are situated in the front and base of the neck. The thyroid gland is the largest and is the controller of growth and metabolism in the body through the secretion of thyroxine.

Metabolism refers to the speed with which the body burns and utilises its cells, and the thyroid stimulates the rate of use of all body tissues except the brain and lymph tissues. It is also the storage site in the body for iodine.

The parathyroid glands are minute glands that are embedded in the connective tissue of the thyroid gland and number between three and ten. They secrete a hormone that regulates the calcium levels in the blood and the tissue fluid.

Hyperthyroidism

This refers to a hyper or overactive thyroid, where too much hormone is produced. This results in loss of weight, rapid heartbeat, nervousness and anxiety. In extreme cases it leads to prominent eyes and a swelling in the neck called a goitre.

Hypothyroidism

This is much more common than hyperthyroidism and refers to an underactive thyroid, which results in weight gain, a dry, flaky skin, lack of energy and a general sluggishness and lack of concentration. Many women especially have mild symptoms of hypothyroidism and yet blood tests show that their hormonal levels are within the normal range.

VRT and reflexology can help to stimulate and balance the thyroid gland if it is under- or over-producing.

The adrenal or supradrenal glands

These are situated on the top of each kidney but have a totally separate function to the kidneys. Each gland has an outer portion called the cortex, which is essential to life as it synthesises over 30 different steroids. The cortex releases sex hormones into the body and also aldosterone, which regulates much of the mineral and water content of the body by stimulating the kidneys. The medulla

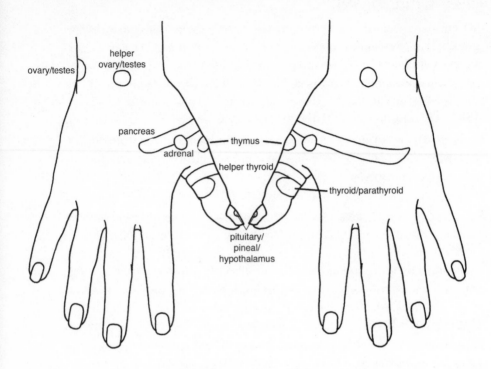

Endocrine reflexes on the hand

plays an important role in stimulating the sympathetic nervous system, as it releases adrenalin and noradrenalin into the body to help it respond to threatening situations.

The pancreas

This contains the islets of Langerhans, which are the hormonal part of the pancreas. The pancreas is also part of the digestive system (see page 142) as it produces digestive enzymes. The islets of Langerhans secrete insulin, which regulates the level of blood sugar and converts its heat into energy. Insulin converts glucose to glycogen and aids the synthesis of DNA and RNA.

The ovaries and testes

These are also part of the reproductive system (see Chapter 18). The ovaries produce the female hormones oestrogen and progesterone, and the testes manufacture sperm and contain cells that manufacture testosterone, the hormone that produces the male characteristics.

How VRT can help

VRT, and reflexology in general, help to balance the body by triggering the organs and glands to work to their optimum ability. Many hormonal conditions can be effectively helped by VRT, especially if self-help on the hands is applied daily. The new nail-working techniques enable you and the client to work very accurately at pinpointing a reflex that requires extra stimulation. The endocrine system is particularly responsive to VRT nail-working and it is recommended that an Endocrine Flush is given in most treatments to balance the body. Diabetics can benefit from a holistic treatment, and couples trying to conceive, as well as pregnant and menopausal women, can all benefit from VRT. Regular treatments are often necessary over a two- to three-month period before deep-seated improvements are observed.

Stress

Overwork or stress can trigger the body to continually produce too much adrenalin, leading to adrenal exhaustion. The adrenal hormones increase the metabolic rate and make a person more alert so that they can deal with a 'flight-or-fight' situation. At times of prolonged stress excessive adrenalin is produced. Regular reflexology is very successful in reducing tension in all ages and all situations. Many illnesses are stress-related, and regular VRT and self-help treatments can enable the body to relax and recover.

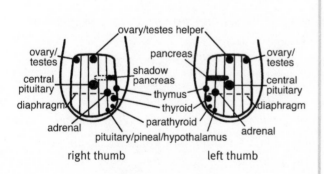

Nail reflexes for stress

VRT techniques and priority reflexes

Condition Stress.

Main reflexes Diaphragm/solar plexus, adrenals and pituitary, and areas most affected.

Synergistic reflexes Solar plexus and area most affected.

Zonal Trigger Adrenals.

Diaphragm Rocking Three minutes.

VRT treatment

- Work every nail zone by zone on the passive hands.
- Use relaxation techniques and basic VRT – Spinal Twist and vigorous tapping.

- Use Whole Body Brush/Lymphatic Stimulation/Diaphragm Rocking. Each can be repeated twice within a treatment.
- To end use Endocrine Flush – work one hand at a time while nail-on-nail to the pituitary reflex.
- Locate the neural pathway for the adrenal.
- Use Knuckle Dusting and Palming.
- To balance, simultaneously hold central nail pituitary reflexes for 30 seconds.
- Use the Harmoniser to finish.

Self-help VRT Apply an Endocrine Flush in every treatment. Hold your right thumbnail on the left thumbnail on the passive hand when in stressful situations, and then repeat on the other hand. Similarly, work the passive and weight-bearing adrenal reflexes when under stress to calm your system or, when you are tired, to boost your system.

Optional complementary help

- **Herbal medicine** Chamomile or lemon-balm tea is an effective relaxant. St John's Wort is helpful in mild depression, but check with your GP if you are on medication, as it can be contraindicated.
- **Homeopathy** Arnica is prescribed for immediate shock but Ignatia 30c is helpful for bereavement, and students taking exams can benefit from Aconite. Picric ac. 30c is helpful for overwork.
- **Hypnotherapy** Tapes are available to aid stress – from basic relaxation tapes to those specially targeted at conditions such as bereavement, fear, loss or guilt. Professional one-to-one help is often beneficial.
- **Massage** This therapy can help to relax tense muscles. The application of aromatherapy oils such as lavender can help to bring about a more balanced state of body and mind. Indian Head Massage can also be very helpful.
- **Nutrition** A lack of essential nutrients can cause symptoms of stress and anxiety. Avoid excessive sugar, caffeine, alcohol, cigarettes or tranquillisers. Adopt a healthy diet and seek advice on appropriate vitamin and mineral supplements for avoiding stress.
- **Phytobiophysics** Certain remedies can be prescribed to target reactions to particular situations and negative states of mind. Up to six formulas at once can be prescribed.
- **Psychotherapy** Can help the root causes of anxiety and tension. Short-term counselling can also help.

Chapter 17

The sense organs

The eyes

The eyes are among the body's most vital and complex organs. They are protected by bone and fatty tissue in the orbital cavity of the skull, and the optic nerve supplies the information to and from the brain. They use only six muscles and rotate on three axes: vertical, horizontal and oblique. They depend on the circulation of blood, lymph and nerve messages just like any other organ in the body. The eye has three layers of tissue: the tough outside layer is the sclera and cornea, which bend the light rays; the middle vascular layer includes the iris, which regulates the amount of light that enters; and the inner layer is the retina, upon which the lens adjusts the focus. The retina can be easily damaged and can become detached. For lubrication and cleansing purposes the eyes are continually bathed with fluid from the tear ducts.

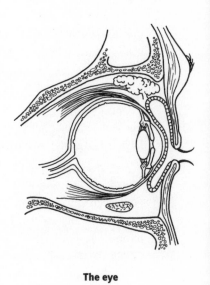

The eye

The skin

The skin has two layers that protect the body: the dermis and the epidermis.

The dermis

The dermis is the unseen fatty, tough part of the skin and is composed of collagen and elastic fibres. All the lymph and blood vessels, hair roots, follicles and glands are contained in the dermis. The nerve endings send messages back to the spinal cord and on to the brain, providing vital information about temperature and the environment. We perspire through our skin and the sweat glands – which are concentrated in the feet, groin and armpits – are also situated in the dermis.

The epidermis

The epidermis is the superficial layer of skin that comes into contact with the outside world. It is the protective layer that covers the nerve endings and sebaceous glands and prevents water and foreign bodies penetrating it, unless it is injured or perforated in some way. Hair and perspiration pass through the epidermis. The epidermis is the barometer regarding our general health and, although it is the superficial part of our bodies, it reflects what is going on internally.

The tongue

The tongue helps us to taste, swallow and speak. It is a voluntary muscle that is covered in papillae, which contain the 9,000 taste buds that are situated mainly at the back of the tongue. These taste buds recognise four basic tastes: salty, bitter, sweet and sour, and the tongue's role when consuming food is to relay the chemical content to the brain through nerve impulses. To gather all the information that the body requires for safe consumption of food, it works closely in conjunction with the eyes and the nose. The tongue is also essential to speech.

The ears

The ears are a complex, three-part mechanism that not only provides the means to hear but also gives balance to the entire body. The external ear – the part that is attached to the side of the head – is called the auricle, and its function is to collect sound waves and conduct them to the external auditory canal, which also contains the glands that secrete wax.

The middle ear is called the tympanic cavity (eardrum), and it is here that the sound is amplified. The sound waves hit the eardrum and the bones in the middle ear, known as the anvil, hammer and stirrup, magnify the vibration. The Eustachian (auditory) tube is a narrow tube that connects the middle ear with the nasopharynx to ensure that the air pressure in the middle ear is the same as the atmospheric pressure. The inner ear or labyrinth is concerned with the equilibrium or balance of the body, and transmits vibrations to the cochlea, which is the essential organ of hearing. It is the channel that transmits information to the brain via the eighth cranial nerve.

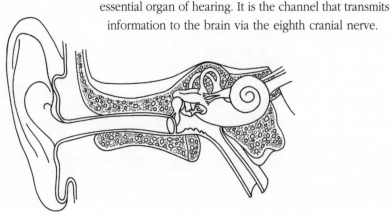

The ear

The nose

This organ, part of the respiratory system, controls the sense of smell. Air inhaled through the nose is filtered and warmed before it reaches the lungs. The nose is lined with a hairy mucous membrane containing blood vessels which are close to the surface. There are three pairs of sinuses which branch out from the nasal passages and go into the skull. Nasal infections can sometimes spread into the sinuses and also into the entire respiratory system. The nose is able to recognise thousands of different smells and relays the information to the brain by special sensory receptors that are found in the nasal cavity.

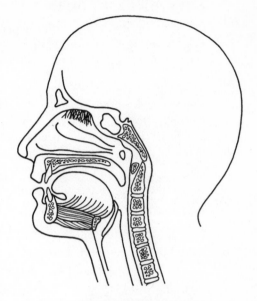

Nasal passages and mouth

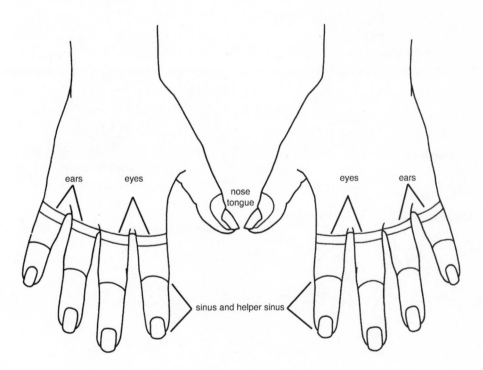

The sense organ reflexes on the hands

How VRT can help

VRT and hand reflexology are extremely effective in pinpointing and treating the sense organs. The eye, ear, nose and tongue reflexes are all situated on the fingers and thumbs.

VRT nail-work allows the therapist to work very specifically. There are minute reflexes around the big toe and thumb that relate to the nose and mouth, and which respond especially well to the firm pressure of VRT on the weight-bearing hand. The skin can sometimes become a little blemished when a person begins a series of reflexology treatments as the body will be stimulated to throw off toxins and the skin is one of the main vehicles of elimination.

Earache

Earache can affect anyone but is most common in children and babies. It is usually caused by inflammation of the middle ear (otitis media) or the Eustachian tube when a blockage of nasal fluid becomes infected. Symptoms include a severe, throbbing pain, pus or wax draining from the ear, a high temperature, partial deafness and often a headache. Glue ear, air-pressure changes on an aircraft and injuries can also cause earache.

VRT techniques and priority reflexes

Condition Earache.

Main reflexes All toes, cervical spine, eyes, ears, adrenals.

Synergistic reflexes Cervical spine, adrenals.

Zonal Trigger Ears.

Diaphragm Rocking Two minutes.

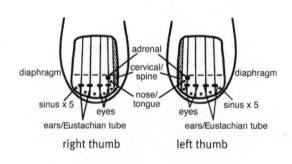

Nail reflexes for earache

VRT treatment

Start with relaxation techniques and basic VRT. Work the lymphatic reflexes three times.

- Use Diaphragm Rocking.
- To end use full Fingertip Pressure to work all ear and eye reflexes as well as the thumbs.
- Locate the neural pathway for the ears. Work both toes to ascertain the most tender cervical reflex.
- Use Knuckle Dusting.
- Nail-working – work the ear reflexes on the thumbnail and secondary nails in zones 4 and 5.
- Use the Harmoniser to finish.

Self-help VRT As above, and specifically stimulate the ear reflexes on the bases of the fourth and fifth fingers on the affected side throughout the day. Work all five nail zones on the thumbs and on the fourth and little fingernails.

Optional complementary help

- **Homeopathy** Belladonna potency 6 is a highly effective and fast-acting remedy, and homeopaths prescribe it for everyone including small children and babies.
- **Indian head massage** This therapy can generally help to soothe the head/ear area. Gentle pressure is applied to the head combined with massage on the head, neck and ear areas.
- **Massage** Some masseurs apply special techniques to the ear and jawbone areas to help keep the Eustachian tube clear.
- **Nutrition** Vitamins and minerals may be prescribed to build up the immune system.
- **Osteopathy** Cranial osteopathy may help to release minute bones in the skull that allow drainage. This can be very helpful for treating glue ear.

Chapter 18

The reproductive system

The reproductive system in women consists of the breasts (mammary glands), two ovaries, two Fallopian tubes, uterus, cervix, vagina, and external genitalia. In men, the reproductive organs comprise the testes, seminal vesicles, vas deferens, prostate and penis. The ovaries and testes also form part of the endocrine or hormonal system.

Female reproductive system

The breasts

The breasts consist of 15 to 20 milk-producing glands embedded in fatty tissue, which supply milk to nourish babies. During pregnancy hormonal changes take place in the breasts and prolactin and oxytocin are secreted, which results in breast milk being produced. Men also have breasts but they are undeveloped.

The ovaries

The ovaries are also part of the endocrine system (see page 150), and are the female reproductive glands. A female is born with about 40,000 eggs in her ovaries and from puberty, when she begins menstruating, until the menopause at about 50 years, she will produce one egg a month. At the mid-monthly cycle the egg

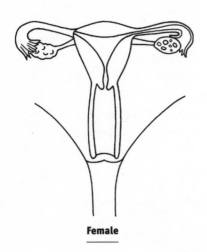

Female

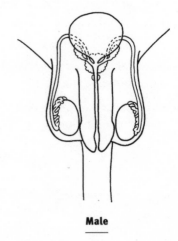

Male

The reproductive system

travels down the Fallopian tube (or uterine tube) and, if it is not fertilised in this tube by a male sperm, the lining of the uterus is shed two weeks later as the monthly period. The pituitary gland controls the function of the ovaries and the hypothalamus also plays a role in stimulating the secretion of hormones that play vital roles in the monthly cycle.

The uterus

This is a muscular organ in which a baby develops. It is situated in the middle of the pelvis, with the bladder in front and the rectum behind. The top of the uterus is called the fundus, the middle is called the body and the lowest part is called the cervix. If fertilisation does not take place, the lining (endometrium) of the uterus is shed each month when the menstrual period commences. The cervix leads into the vagina, which is a hollow, muscular organ that connects the uterus to the external genitalia, which include the vulva and clitoris. The vagina is extremely elastic and is capable of expanding to receive the male penis and also in childbirth, when it becomes the birth canal as the baby passes from the uterus into the outside world.

Male reproductive system

The testes

The testes are two male sex glands that descend from the abdominal cavity while the baby is still in the womb and, by the eighth month, have reached the external pouch of skin called the scrotum. The testicles produce the hormone testosterone as well as sperm, which mature for three weeks in the epididymis, a coiled tube lying around the testes. Each sex gland is attached to the body by a single cord called the vas deferens (sperm ducts), which contains a number of nerves and blood vessels. The sperm then travels to the seminal vesicles, which produce seminal fluid. When a man has an orgasm the sperm passes into the urethra and is ejaculated with the seminal fluid. The bladder and testicles share the same exit, the 20 cm urethra that runs the length of the penis. There is a muscular action that prevents urine and seminal fluids being passed at the same time.

The prostate gland

This is a cluster of small glands which surround the urethra at the point where it joins the bladder. There is debate about the actual function of the prostate and it is suggested that it provides additional secretions into the seminal fluid to help the active movement of the sperm. Many men's prostate glands begin to enlarge and stiffen after the age of 45 and in later life this can put pressure on the urethra. The first sign of prostate trouble is a weakened flow of urine with an urgent need to pass water at night, although the flow and contents passed are low.

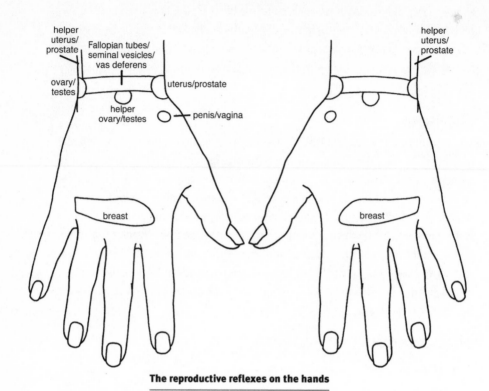

The reproductive reflexes on the hands

The penis

The male sex organ consists of spongy tissue full of minute blood vessels which become engorged when the man is sexually aroused, causing it to become erect and increase in size. A single ejaculation contains millions of sperm, only one of which is required to fertilise the female egg. The penis consists of involuntary muscles and elongated masses of erectile tissue and surrounds the urethra, which transports the semen and urine. The tip of the penis is referred to as the glans and is covered by a loose hood of skin called the foreskin. In the centre of the glans is a slit from which urine and semen is discharged. This is called the external urethral orifice.

How VRT can help

VRT and reflexology appear to help the body regulate its hormonal output and this can be particularly beneficial to women in puberty, during conception, in child-bearing and at the menopause. There are reflexes connected to every part of the reproductive system and reflexology has a major role to play in prostate problems in men and sexual difficulties in both sexes. VRT on the hands and feet can be quickly applied to a woman in labour if she is able to stand.

Menopausal problems

The menopause is not an illness but a period of physical and emotional change which affects some women more than others. A change in the monthly cycle is usually the first indicator that the balance between the ovaries, hypothalamus and pituitary glands is changing.

Many women experience heavy periods or even flooding. Regular treatments appear to help regulate the menstrual cycle and temper some of the adverse symptoms such as heavy periods, mood swings and hot flushes. Genital symptoms, such as loss of tone and elasticity of vaginal, uterine and urethral tissues, are common. Reflexology and VRT aim to help alleviate the symptoms holistically, as well as by treating specific reflexes.

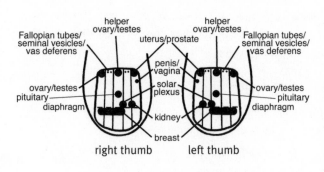

Nail reflexes for menopausal problems

> **VRT techniques and priority reflexes**
>
> **Condition** Menopausal problems.
>
> **Main reflexes** All glands, diaphragm, solar plexus, kidneys, uterus, breast.
>
> **Synergistic reflexes** Uterus/prostate, thyroid.
>
> **Zonal Trigger** Pituitary.

VRT treatment

Start with several minutes of relaxation techniques and basic VRT, as well as concentrated work on the lumbar spine (including Spinal Twist) and abdominal area. See the illustration on page 153 for all endocrine reflexes.

- Use Lymphatic Stimulation for one minute per hand and Diaphragm Rocking.
- Use the Whole Body Brush.
- To end use Palmar Pressure technique.
- Locate the uterus neural pathway reflex (L3) and connect with Zonal Trigger. In severe cases two endocrine neural pathway reflexes could be worked within the same treatment.
- Use Palming – concentrate on the small and large intestines. Work across the transverse colon reflex.

- Nail-work on the thumbs using connecting techniques and the Endocrine or Reproductive Flush including the pituitary and uterus reflex.
- For flooding problems connect the Zonal Trigger to the uterus reflex and work the pituitary nail reflex.
- Work ovary and helper reflexes simultaneously.
- Use the Harmoniser to finish.
- Show the client three priority reflexes, usually pituitary, uterus and ovary, to work on the weight-bearing hand twice daily between treatments.

Self-help VRT Work the pituitary nail reflex whenever a hot flush occurs by holding each thumb, nail-on-nail, for up to 45 seconds. For lack of libido in women use the Whole Body Brush several times per day, using the knuckles to work the Fallopian tube/vas deferens and Zonal Triggers, plus pituitary and ovaries. For painful periods pinch the passive hand uterus reflexes on the palm and dorsum at the same time and hold for 30 seconds.

Optional complementary help

- **Applied Kinesiology** This therapy can help to balance the body hormonally and clients can be tested for suitable remedies.
- **Aromatherapy** Many oils are helpful, especially geranium, rose and clary sage, but professional advice should be sought.
- **Herbal medicine** Hormonal disturbances can respond well to wild yam or agnus castus, and specific herbal formulas are available in health shops targeted at premenstrual tension and the menopause. For best results consult a professional herbalist.
- **Homeopathy** Many remedies are effective, such as Sepia and Pulsatilla for period problems, and Lachesis for hot flushes.
- **Nutrition** A diet rich in plant oestrogens, found in foods like soya and tofu, helps to lessen the menopausal effects. Star Flower and Evening Primrose oil appear to help premenstrual tension.
- **Phytobiophysics** There are remedies that help balance the body and specific remedies that help women's hormonal problems. A specialised practitioner will test for the correct formula.

Chapter 19

Summary

Having read this book you will have discovered that VRT for hands is a simple but extremely effective therapy. Nothing could be easier than discreetly working your hands to help you sleep, to aid digestion, to cure a headache or to calm you in stressful situations. Your hands are a window into your body, and by learning to apply VRT and conventional hand reflexology you will be able to tap into your body's own natural healing properties. There is no need to feel you have to particularly believe in a certain response to get results. You are simply adopting a pragmatic approach to health by triggering reflexes in your body, which then enable it to help itself.

Pressure points on the hands and feet were discovered 5,000 years ago and over the centuries the techniques associated with VRT and reflexology have been rediscovered, developed and defined. Babies respond to the gentle healing touch, and the physically impaired and the terminally ill have all gained help and relief from this therapy. Additionally, I and many others have achieved success with clients who have booked a reflexology appointment as a last resort because allopathic medicine or other therapies have failed to help their condition. And it can be a rewarding experience to treat a sceptical partner, colleague or family member of a client. These people often arrive very unwillingly because someone has made them come! In most cases they are agreeably surprised with the physical improvements and the experience of total relaxation.

Summary of VRT hand techniques

Below is a summary of all the VRT techniques you have learnt in this book. This is your VRT tool box and, used wisely and with discernment, it will allow you to treat your clients and yourself. It will also enable you to teach the rudiments of VRT to your family, friends and clients, which will allow them to accelerate their recovery and give them more control over their health and general well-being.

Basic VRT

Basic VRT Sequence This treats all reflexes three-dimensionally via the dorsum (top) of the hand, and should be used in all treatments except first aid, when only the wrists and spinal reflexes are worked to prime the body.

Synergistic reflexology Increases the powerful response on two priority conditions by working the hand and foot reflexes simultaneously. Limited to three reflexes.

Zonal Triggers Increases the powerful response further on the top-priority condition by working three reflexes simultaneously. Limit: one priority reflex or occasionally two priority reflexes within the same bodily system. There are options for working the three reflexes on the hands, on the feet, or on the hands and feet when synergistic reflexology is introduced.

Harmoniser An extremely important technique that should be used at least once in every treatment. It has been developed to balance and consolidate a treatment. It also appears to prevent over-reaction to a treatment or the possibility of a healing crisis occurring. It can be repeated frequently during a treatment if necessary.

Self-help Harmoniser To administer self-help, or to calm yourself down. Can be used on the passive or weight-bearing hands.

Pituitary Pinch This technique helps to consolidate the treatment by balancing the endocrine system.

Diaphragm Rocking Diaphragm Rocking aids relaxation and helps to combat insomnia. It is a profound technique that allows the body to prioritise and channel a healing stimulus to the area most in need. It also enables the reflexologist to be energised during a session, as it appears to allow a neutral exchange of energy between the therapist and the client.

Advanced VRT

Lymphatic Stimulation This helps to cleanse and stimulate the abdominal area but can be used as a general boost for the immune system and for those suffering from oedema.

Knuckle Dusting A stimulating technique that helps treat the entire body. It is particularly useful for asthma and mild depression, and for stimulating the nervous system.

Palming A firm and calming move that is useful for shoulder problems and other conditions where the reflexes are situated on the metacarpal bones.

Palmar Pressure The heel of the weight-bearing hand is raised from the flat surface so that more pressure is put on the upper metacarpal bones. This is a useful technique for working the dorsum of the hand.

Fingertip Pressure A unique way of working the splayed weight-bearing fingers and thumbs. It is particularly useful for treating head, neck and sinus conditions.

Neural pathway reflexes A profound and precise working of the spinal nerve reflexes using the knuckles rather than the fingertips.

Neural pathways, Zonal Triggers The combination of three points worked simultaneously on the hand or foot (rather than the hand and foot as in synergistic reflexology) increases the power and stimulus to an area. The result is that a certain organ, gland or part of the skeletal system can be more precisely targeted if the body has not responded to synergistic reflexology and the Zonal Trigger.

Whole Body Brush The knuckles or fingertips are used to work around the wrist Zonal Triggers, then pinch and brush the dorsum (top) of the hand from the wrist to the fingertips.

VRT nail-working

The basic VRT nail-working technique involves pressing the thumb or fingernail tip onto the nail. The aim is to work the nail reflexes on a grid system of five zones per nail, preferably when the hand is weight-bearing.

Embarking on hand reflexology

The various VRT hand reflexology techniques listed above can be considered to be part of the tool box of skills you will need to be a successful practitioner. Dwight Byers, President of the International Institute of Reflexology, likens reflexologists to mechanics. Once they have completed their training they have an adequate tool box and, as they take postgraduate courses, the number of tools grows larger. However, it is important to use discernment when treating a client. Not all the tools will be suitable at any one time, and different techniques will be necessary as the treatments progress over the weeks.

You must be careful not to overwork the reflexes, especially when they are in the weight-bearing position. VRT is very powerful and therefore working any reflex should be limited to 30 seconds, although you can return to it during the five-minute VRT treatment to stimulate it for a few extra seconds, as long as the pressure is not continuous.

When treating the passive hands there is another consideration: if someone had a painful hip, for example, that area on the hands and the connecting spinal reflexes should be worked for perhaps ten minutes in total on both hands to really trigger the reflex response. It is not appropriate to just work the shoulder reflexes for a few minutes and spend an equal time on all the parts of the hands. You need to address the priority condition.

Share your skills with discernment

You may be fully trained as a VRT practitioner or be someone who has learnt a few general VRT skills for use on family and friends. In both cases, be prepared to offer help where it is needed, but also respect another person's boundaries and remember that not everyone enthusiastically embraces complementary care, especially if it is suddenly offered to them in a public setting. I once treated a woman who told me she had been put off reflexology years before because a well-meaning reflexologist had embarrassed her by insisting on working on her feet at a party as she happened to mention that she had a headache. Discernment is key to helping other people and their privacy must always be respected.

Ask your clients and friends to do their homework!

You can help your clients to help themselves by applying a few VRT weight-bearing techniques to the hands for a few minutes twice daily. VRT is a powerful therapy that responds effectively to the amateur touch. I suggest that you photo-copy the hand chart on page 25 and give it to each client, with the wrist and three priority reflexes highlighted. Show them how to work their weight-bearing hand on rising and before bed each day for two to three minutes each time. When using VRT, reflexologists often report a 60 to 70 per cent improvement in symptoms over a short period, but I am convinced that this result can be improved on with daily self-help VRT on the hands (see Appendix 2).

The hands are just as responsive to VRT as the feet and are much more acces-sible when it comes to giving a treatment. Many people who would not allow their feet to be worked due to embarrassment or sensitivity are often very willing to offer their hands to a professional reflexologist using advanced VRT techniques, or to a layperson's quick VRT basic treatment. Everyone can benefit from self-help VRT which, like many complementary therapies, can trigger the wonderful innate power of the body to help heal itself.

Guide to treating common ailments with VRT

How to use this chart

This reference chart can be used for all types of VRT treatment.

1. Select the condition and work the entire hand in the usual way using basic VRT, but briefly concentrate on the areas mentioned under Main reflexes to be worked, or change the order of priority depending on need. During the conventional part of the treatment you can return again to work these priority areas on the passive hands.

2. At the end of a treatment, whether it lasts five or 35 minutes, return to the reflexes of the wrists on the weight-bearing hands. Work the wrists and brush across the Zonal Triggers.

3. Select the two synergistic reflexes listed and work the corresponding hand and foot reflexes at the same time. Repeat on the other hand.

4. Select the priority reflex on the dorsum (top) of the hand and hold. Find the corresponding reflex on the foot and work around the bracelet of the ankle carefully until you locate the relevant Zonal Trigger. Link the reflex and Zonal Trigger and relocate the corresponding reflex on the client's hand. Hold all three for 30 seconds and repeat on the other hand and foot.

5. Diaphragm Rocking should, ideally, be used during every treatment, including the five-minute basic VRT, and 15 rocks per hand should be the minimum. In some cases, it is appropriate to rock the hands for much longer to allow the energy to be pumped to the priority area in the body. These instructions are given in the Zonal Triggers column.

6. Advanced and nail-working techniques can be selected from your repertoire and added to your treatment. See Chapters 4 and 5.

7. Basic VRT can take up to five minutes at the beginning of a treatment, but usually takes less. At the end of the session swiftly work the wrists and spinal reflexes before selecting some advanced techniques to use for up to five minutes. Always conclude with the Harmoniser.

Condition	Main reflexes to be worked	Synergistic reflexes	Zonal Triggers (DR = Diaphragm Rocking)
Acne	Liver, all glands, colon, kidneys	Adrenals/colon	Liver
Alcoholism	Liver, pancreas, diaphragm, brain, solar plexus	Brain/pancreas	Liver DR 3 minutes
Anaemia	Spleen, liver	Liver	Spleen
Angina	Heart (ankle reflex), heart/lung, diaphragm, sigmoid colon, thoracic calf points	Sigmoid colon/diaphragm	Heart/lung DR 2 minutes
Arthritis	Entire foot, spine, adrenals, kidneys, areas most affected	Spine, adrenals	Area most affected
Asthma	Diaphragm, chest/lung, bronchials, ileocecal valve, adrenals	Bronchials, adrenals	Chest/lung DR 2 to 3 minutes
Backache	Full spine, neck/shoulder, pelvic/sciatic	Pelvic sciatic/neck, shoulder	Appropriate spinal reflex
Bedwetting	Whole spine, diaphragm	Bladder/adrenals	Lumbar spine DR 2 minutes
Cataracts	Eyes/ears, pituitary gland, cervical spine, kidneys	Cervical spine, kidneys	Ears/eyes
Colds and flu	Sinus, diaphragm, chest/lung, bronchials, ileocecal valve, adrenals, thyroid gland, lymphatics and ears/eyes	Bronchials/sinus	Lymphatics DR 2 minutes
Coughs	Chest/lung, throat, lymphatics	Throat, chest/lung	Lymphatics
Constipation	Large intestine, liver and gall bladder, adrenals, ileocecal valve, lumbar spine, adrenals	Lower spine, liver	Colon DR 2 minutes
Cystitis	Bladder, kidneys, ureters, lumbar spine, adrenals	Lumbar spine, ureters	Bladder
Diabetes	Pancreas, all glands, liver	Liver and thyroid	Pancreas
Depression	Solar plexus, diaphragm, pituitary, neck, adrenals, brain (work all toes)	Solar plexus, pituitary	Brain DR 2 minutes
Diarrhoea	Small intestine, large intestine, lumbar spine, solar plexus, ileocecal valve, liver, adrenals	Lumbar spine, liver	Colon
Drug addiction	Solar plexus, diaphragm, adrenals, thyroid, pituitary, brain, liver, kidneys, work all toes	Liver, kidneys	Brain DR 3 minutes
Earache	All toes, cervical spine, eyes/ears, adrenals	Adrenals, cervical spine	Eyes/ears
Eczema	Lymphatics, adrenals, intestines, kidneys, solar plexus, pituitary, areas most affected	Area most affected, kidneys	Lymphatics DR 3 minutes
Eye problems	Ears/eyes, kidneys, cervical spine, all toes, neck	Cervical spine, kidneys	Ears/eyes
Fainting	Heart, brain, pituitary and cervical spine	Heart and brain	Pituitary DR 2–3 minutes

Condition	Main reflexes to be worked	Synergistic reflexes	Zonal Triggers (DR = Diaphragm Rocking)
Fatigue	Diaphragm, solar plexus, heart, all glands, brain, spleen, spine	Pituitary, adrenals	Solar plexus DR 2 to 3 minutes
Fever	Pituitary, thyroid, cervical spine	Thyroid, cervical spine	Pituitary
Gall stones	Liver and gall bladder, thyroid, solar plexus, diaphragm	Thyroid, liver	Gall bladder
Glandular fever	Lymphatics, spleen, pituitary, diaphragm, solar plexus, areas most affected, i.e. glands or neck	Area most affected, pituitary	Lymphatics
Hangover	Liver, head/brain, kidney	Head/brain, kidney	Liver DR 2 minutes
Hayfever	Head, throat, sinuses, eyes, adrenals	Adrenals, throat	Sinuses
Headache	Head, cervical and lumbar spine, solar plexus, small and large intestines, liver	Cervical spine, intestines	Head DR 2 to 3 minutes
Heartburn/ Indigestion	Diaphragm, stomach, solar plexus, oesophagus	Diaphragm, oesophagus	Stomach DR 2 minutes
Haemorrhoids	Large intestine, rectum, lumbar spine	Large intestine, lumber spine	Rectum
Hernia – abdominal	Large intestine, groin, adrenals, spinal reflexes	Adrenals, large intestine	Groin
Hiatus Hernia	Diaphragm, adrenals, stomach, chest/lung	Diaphragm, adrenals	Stomach
Hip problems	Lumbar spine, hip/knee, sciatic, shoulder (referred pain link)	Sciatic, lumbar spine	Hip/knee
Hypertension (high blood pressure)	Kidneys, diaphragm, solar plexus, all glands, heart	Kidneys, heart	Diaphragm DR 2 minutes
Hypotension (low blood pressure)	Diaphragm, solar plexus, all glands, heart, thyroid, kidneys	Kidneys, heart	Diaphragm DR 2 minutes
Impotence	All glands, reproductive organs, spinal reflexes, diaphragm, brain	Brain, reproductive organs	Testes DR 3 minutes
Incontinence	Bladder, kidneys, ureters, lumbar spine, solar plexus, diaphragm	Lumbar spine, solar plexus	Ureter/bladder junction
Infertility	All glands, diaphragm, solar plexus, lumbar spine, brain, uterus	Thyroid, lumbar spine	Ovary/testes DR 3 minutes
Insomnia	All toes, cervical spine, neck, shoulder, pituitary/pineal gland, solar plexus, brain	Solar plexus, pituitary/ pineal	Brain DR – 3 minutes
Irritable Bowel Syndrome	Intestines, solar plexus, diaphragm, adrenals, lumbar spine	Lumbar spine, adrenals	Large intestine
Jet lag	Diaphragm, pituitary/ hypothalamus, neck, brain, solar plexus	Brain, neck	Pituitary/hypothalamus DR 3 minutes

Condition	Main reflexes to be worked	Synergistic reflexes	Zonal Triggers (DR = Diaphragm Rocking)
Knee problems	Hip/knee reflexes, lumbar spine sciatic. Work the elbow (referral area)	Lumbar spine, sciatic	Hip/knee reflexes
ME – myalgic encephalitis and post-viral syndrome	Brush reflexes for a maximum of 30 seconds–1 minute each hand for first 3 treatments. All glands, lymphatics, spleen, solar plexus/diaphragm, areas most affected, head	Lymphatics, adrenals	Head DR 3 minutes
Menopause/ hot flushes	All glands, diaphragm, solar plexus, kidneys, uterus	Pituitary, uterus	Thyroid
Menstrual pain	Fallopian tubes, lumbar spine, uterus, all glands, diaphragm, solar plexus	Ovary, lumbar spine	Uterus
Migraine	Head, eyes, stomach, cervical and lumbar spine, solar plexus, intestines, liver	Stomach, cervical spine	Head
Multiple sclerosis	Diaphragm, solar plexus, spine, brain, all glands	Solar plexus, brain	Spine
Neck problems	Neck, cervical spine, lumbar spine, shoulder	Neck, shoulder	Spine
Oedema	Lymphatics, kidneys, adrenals, leg reflex, hand referral area for swollen foot	Kidneys, adrenals	Lymphatics
PMT	Solar plexus, all glands, affected areas, e.g. abdomen or uterus	Pituitary, solar plexus	Area most affected
Pregnancy	Brush all reflexes lightly in first three months. Then work solar plexus, uterus, all glands, bladder, adrenals, lumbar spine	Pituitary, lumbar spine	Solar plexus
Sciatica	Diaphragm, solar plexus, lower lumbar spine, sciatic, shoulder, hip/knee	Lower lumbar spine, hip/knee	Sciatic
Shoulder problems	Shoulder, arm, thoracic spine, diaphragm	Arm, thoracic spine	Shoulder
Shingles	Lung, chest, lymphatics, affected area, adrenals, pituitary, thyroid	Lymphatics, thyroid	Affected area
Sinus problems	Sinuses, ileocecal valve, ears, eyes, Eustachian tube, Cervical spine	Eustacian tube, Cervical spine	Sinus (find most tender reflex on thumb or finger)
Skin problems	Solar plexus, diaphragm, intestines, thyroid, kidneys, pituitary, affected area	Thyroid, solar plexus	Intestines DR 2 minutes
Sore throat	Throat/neck, lymphatics, adrenals, solar plexus	Lymphatics	Throat/neck
Travel sickness and nausea	Stomach, adrenals, head, thoracic spine, lymphatics	Head, lymphatics	Stomach
Stress	Diaphragm, solar plexus, adrenals, pituitary, areas most affected	Area most affected, solar plexus	Adrenals

Condition	Main reflexes to be worked	Synergistic reflexes	Zonal Triggers (DR = Diaphragm Rocking)
Stroke	Toes, reflexes to affected areas, whole spine, dorsal wrist reflexes	Affected areas and dorsal wrist reflex	Brain. Work thumb tips, especially alternate side from paralysis.
Thyroid – under or over-active	Thyroid, pituitary, adrenal, eyes, cervical spine	Pituitary, cervical spine	Thyroid
Tinnitus	Ears, sinuses, cervical spine, diaphragm, solar plexus, adrenals	Cervical spine, sinuses	Ears
Toothache	Toes, below nail of big toe, adrenals, cervical spine	Adrenals, cervical spine	Below nail of big toe
Tonsillitis	Lymphatics, toes, cervical spine, adrenals	Lymphatics, cervical spine	Between end of nail and first joint on the thumb
Tumours	Whole spine, all glands, solar plexus, areas most affected	Pituitary, solar plexus	Area most affected
Ulcers – external	Diaphragm, solar plexus, lymphatics, areas most affected, adrenals	Stomach, lymphatics	Duodenum
Ulcers – internal	Stomach, duodenum, diaphragm, solar plexus, lymphatics	Lymphatics, solar plexus	Area most affected
Varicose veins	Liver, heart reflex on dorsal ankle, intestines, adrenals, legs, arm as referral area	Liver, adrenals	Legs
Whiplash	Cervical spine, all toes, adrenals, shoulder, neck, lumbar spine	Between thumb and index finger, shoulder	Cervical spine

VRT and reflexology in the workplace

In recent years many employers have been taking a more holistic view of the benefits they can give to their staff than has been the case in the past. Some may offer a pension package, medical insurance, subsidised canteen or even a crèche, while others are beginning to see the value of preventative health care for their employees. Pragmatic decisions have to be made when it comes to spending company money and many firms now offer complementary therapies to staff at subsidised rates – the resulting reduction in sick leave more than pays for the therapist's fee. It is estimated that 75 per cent of all illness is stress-related and this can substantially reduce productivity and efficiency in the workplace. Prolonged stress can lead to tiredness and irritability, a weakening of the immune system and the development of physical illness. In 1995 there were more than two million cases of work-related illness in the UK alone, which cost the country £16 billion. With VRT and reflexology many conditions, ranging from neck-ache and repetitive strain injury to Irritable Bowel Syndrome and stress, can be treated in a gentle, effective and non-invasive manner.

In Denmark, reflexology is the number one complementary therapy and many large organisations such as Lego, the Danish Post Office and Danish Fisheries employ reflexologists to keep their workforce healthy and reduce the number of staff sick days. In the UK reflexologists now regularly run clinics in industries as diverse as insurance, banking, retail, telecommunications and manufacturing.

The staff are often initially invited to a short presentation by the therapist to introduce them to the concept of reflexology, and then they are offered a brief taster session. Reduced sickness and absenteeism, increased productivity and the attendant financial benefits for the company are the visible results, but many employees experience a positive effect on morale as well as health, and appreciate the individual care and space to discuss matters in confidence.

VRT on the hands and feet has enabled many reflexologists to offer treatments of a shorter duration than a standard reflexology treatment (see Chapter 5), which can be more appropriate in the workplace. Most reflexologists give 45 to 60 minutes of conventional foot reflexology treatments. Conventional hand treatments take 30 to 35 minutes. With VRT, staff are given a few minutes' treatment. They then recline on a chair or couch for conventional reflexology on the hands or feet. At the end of this shorter session advanced VRT techniques are introduced to treat specific conditions. VRT can be particularly useful, for example, in helping many types of postural problems that people tend to suffer from in the work environment. An additional benefit applies to those who have never considered holistic health care before, preferring to take medication from the chemist or their doctor. Subsidised treatments in the workplace introduce them to natural preventive health care in a non-threatening setting – and with the added benefit of being financially viable through subsidisation.

Approaching companies

If you wish to work in a company but do not have a personal contact, you should put together a Curriculum Vitae and presentation package and send it to the Human Resources department. Some professional bodies such as the Association of Reflexologists have put together leaflets and presentation packs on reflexology in the workplace, and it is worth approaching your professional organisation to see what can be bought or hired before you embark on the slow and difficult task of writing your own leaflets. It is usually advisable not only to offer to come and discuss your work with a senior administrator but also to suggest giving a sample treatment to several members of staff as a free taster session. Ensure that the treatment room supplied is satisfactory and well ventilated, with adequate heating. You will need a small table and chair for VRT hand treatments. If you are leaving equipment in the room between clinics, check that the contents of the room are insured, and that the room will be locked when not in use.

Taking case histories

It is very important to take a full case history and this is not really possible when you are offering shortened treatments of only 20 minutes or so. The best solution is to make the first session ten minutes longer, so you can discuss the background to the patient's condition – and, if desired, charge accordingly. Or you can send the client a detailed pro-forma case history questionnaire which can be completed in advance and brought to the first appointment for discussion. The first visit should take 30 minutes and subsequent treatments can be as short as 20 minutes. Despite VRT's success in obtaining quick results it is unethical to offer very short treatments with no time for evaluation, advice or the taking of a case history. I am convinced that no company would take such an offer seriously and it could discourage them from investigating further the real benefits of VRT and reflexology. Five-minute VRT treatments are for family, friends and first aid only.

Confidentiality

This is always paramount when working as a therapist and even more so when you are in a workplace environment, in which colleagues may talk about each other or about confidential company matters. Always seek permission from the individual you are treating before reporting back to senior staff about a condition that appears to be improving or otherwise. It is up to the individual to choose what to reveal to their management.

General health

Encourage patients to drink enough water and to look at their dietary requirements where necessary. The hectic office environment can sometimes dictate a lifestyle where workers rely on machine coffee for an instant caffeine lift and chocolate bars to replace breakfast or lunch. Always remember that every client has to make their own decisions and you should not impose a regime of healthy eating or exercise on anyone.

Self-help VRT

Many clients are grateful to be given a few VRT self-help techniques (see Chapter 6) and it is useful to duplicate the hand chart from this book and mark three or four reflexes that they can work on between treatments.

PRACTITIONER'S CASE STUDY

Condition: Jet lag.

Duration: Two weeks.

Client: Male. **Aged:** 32.

Aim of treatment: To help relieve chronic tiredness due to jet lag following an exhausting business trip to America.

Result: The client slept deeply during session and slept very well that night and was fine next day.

Practitioner's comment: The client now books in within 24 hours of returning from business trips to have his body clock adjusted – and the treatment works every time.

Author's comment: Diaphragm Rocking, which was used during the treatment, is one of the most powerful reflexology techniques. It was originally developed before VRT was discovered, to help in correcting sleep patterns. It is particularly helpful for jet lag, and clients can be taught the VRT self-help Diaphragm Rocking method.

VRT lends itself to the workplace

- VRT and reflexology are particularly useful in the workplace because the therapist can treat the staff member on a couch, chair or even standing up for a short treatment.

- VRT is a gentle, non-invasive therapy, particularly when working on the hands.

- Complete VRT can give a person a fully effective treatment in 20 minutes if necessary.

Feedback from VRT treatments in the workplace

It is always interesting to work in a large organisation as there will be a wide variety of conditions presented by staff. In hospitals many of the nursing staff and carers present a variety of orthopaedic problems, which are often old injuries that get exacerbated by lifting or bending.

The following examples illustrate the variety of ailments that can be quickly and successfully treated within the workplace or office environment. Six members of staff, in a large organisation, were selected for a small survey I conducted in July 2002. None had received reflexology before, and in each case there was a positive response to the treatment within the first one or two weeks. After four weeks some conditions had improved by over 90 per cent. Each patient's 20- to 30-minute treatment began with basic VRT on the feet, then they were treated with conventional reflexology while using the hands synergistically. The client kept a record of their reaction to each treatment, and was given VRT hand charts marked with specific reflexes to treat with self-help VRT twice a day for a few minutes between the weekly treatments. All six results were exceptionally positive and after four treatments both the client and I evaluated the progress made since VRT commenced.

Client A

Client A was a female caterer who had been badly hurt in a car accident seven months previously, resulting in whiplash. She had very restricted and excruciatingly painful neck movements that caused headaches. Her sleep patterns were so disturbed that she barely slept for more than two hours at any one time.
Result Her neck mobility improved by 50 per cent. She can now turn her head from side to side with no pain. There was no lasting improvement for the headaches, but 100 per cent improvement in sleep problems. Her levels of stress and tension were greatly reduced.

Client B

Client B was an administrator in her early forties who suffered from long-term repetitive strain injury. Her shoulder and the right side of the neck were stiff and painful when her hand was held in a lateral position. This had become a chronic condition. She reported painful knees that clicked, possibly due to early signs of arthritis. She also had a sprained right ankle.

Result She felt a 90 per cent improvement in arm, neck and shoulder in terms of reduced pain and increased mobility. Her sprained ankle responded positively to VRT. Her knees did not improve, but she felt she had benefited holistically from the treatments.

Client C

Client C was a manager who had suffered for three weeks from an extremely painful left elbow. His right knee clicked every few days, causing him to experience a momentary excruciating pain when he put pressure on it at a certain angle.

Result His elbow greatly improved from the first treatment and was virtually 100 per cent recovered by the end of four weeks. The clicks in the knee lessened and were not painful when they occurred. He experienced immediate relief for his hurt ankle.

Client D

Client D was a care assistant who had suffered from right lower lumbar back pain for seven to eight months. Her work necessitated standing all day, and as time passed her back became increasingly sore. She had taken two weeks off work at the onset of the pain and a further four weeks off five months later. She also had chronic eczema in her ear, which caused discomfort and irritation.

Result Her back improved considerably over four weeks with little soreness remaining. Her long-term ear problem became worse before it got completely better. Her sleep was much improved.

Client E

Client E was a nurse who had left neck and arm problems. She had limited mobility and could barely raise her arms behind her back. She had badly sprained her left ankle three months previously, had used crutches and then a stick for a while, and was still suffering from weakness and soreness in that area. Her foot was permanently at an awkward angle and she felt she could feel the bones almost grating as she walked.

Result Increased mobility in the arm by the end of the first treatment. She can now stretch her arm straight. After the first treatment she had more backwards arm movement, which has further improved since then. Her long-term problem with the left foot improved – it became virtually pain-free and she found walking easier. However, self-help was not enough and she requires professional VRT treatment to maintain her foot's condition.

Client F

Client F was a manager who had whiplash injury and lower back, hip and neck pain. All these were long-standing problems that occasionally flared up. She was regularly treated by an osteopath.

Result Her neck is now generally much improved but remains a little stiff. Her entire body is much more relaxed than it had been for a considerable period, and her hips are much improved. Her osteopath noted these improvements and suggested a longer gap between treatments for the first time ever. VRT self-help techniques also helped her holistically.

Conclusion

All the staff reported that they felt VRT/reflexology had been of great benefit and said they would continue to use self-help hand reflexology when required.

One person did express doubt that the self-help VRT on the hands would be sufficiently powerful to achieve this level of results without the added input of a full VRT treatment. This is a very valid point as, for example, Client E found self-help VRT was not enough and her foot only improved when I worked her hand. However, the general opinion so far is that when the hands are worked in a weight-bearing position the body is particularly responsive, whether the person has been treated professionally or not.

All work environments need a healthy workforce to function efficiently. VRT and reflexology when used together are a gentle non-invasive therapy that can help to maintain fitness, and to reduce stress and other work-related illnesses.

Reflexology in the workplace

Odense Post Office in Denmark, which has employed a full-time reflexologist since 1990, reports a saving of around £100,000 a year due to a reduction in sickness and absenteeism of 13.3 per cent.

The Human Resources Director of Lego reported at a reflexology conference that his company employed several reflexologists on various sites and treatments were available for all levels of staff. The company felt this was a pragmatic financial decision as the amount paid to the therapists was much less than the productivity and revenue lost through sickness in the years before reflexology was offered.

Ishoj Municipal Health Department recorded 2,499 fewer hours of sick leave over a six-month period in which employees received reflexology. This saved the company £21,490.

Therapies that complement VRT and reflexology

Reflexology and VRT complement most other holistic therapies and, if progress is slow, it is often pertinent to evaluate the situation and perhaps try a different therapy, or combine two. For example, VRT can help to free a stiff neck but the final improvement may come about after a deep tissue massage. It is very important to consult a trained therapist who has received recognised training, is fully insured and belongs to a professional body. Many clients want to be treated by an experienced therapist who is used to dealing with a wide variety of conditions. However, a recently qualified therapist will have the benefit of being well-versed in the latest techniques and research. All reflexologists have to build up their working practice and some will offer reduced fees or include an extra free treatment as an introduction to their work. Influential journals such as *Positive Health* are highly informative and objective about the many complementary therapies on offer, and include information on the latest research. (See Recommended Reading, page 193.)

The following pages give a brief description of the therapies that complement reflexology. The therapies I have selected are personal preferences and it is important to look further than the guidelines given here if you have a specific need or an intransigent problem. For details on how to find VRT practitioners and other holistic therapists, see Useful Addresses, page 191.

It is advisable to let your doctor know that you are undertaking a course of treatment with a complementary practitioner. Many GPs are very sympathetic to complementary medicine and some offer therapies within their practice. Additionally, if you are considering combining more than one complementary therapy, it is essential to inform each practitioner so they can work accordingly. It is important to note that acupuncture and acupressure, while excellent in their own right, are contraindicated with reflexology and should not be combined.

Alexander Technique

This technique is usually taught on a one-to-one basis, and is used to treat a wide range of postural, muscular-skeletal problems, as well as to teach breathing techniques. Teachers of the technique instruct their pupils to mentally inhibit bad physical and postural habits learnt over many years by retargeting messages to the brain and central nervous system.

Applied Kinesiology

Applied Kinesiology was developed by chiropractor Dr George Goodheart in the late 1960s and is a means of assessing imbalances in the body and finding the most effective therapy to resolve them. Muscle response is used to obtain this information from the body. Kinesiologists are taught how to assess your health problems and how to apply appropriate techniques to correct and balance the body's systems. Kinesiology is non-intrusive and addresses all aspects of health: structural, biochemical, emotional and electromagnetic.

Aromatherapy

Aromatherapy involves the use of massage coupled with highly concentrated oils extracted from plants. The essential oils are diluted by being mixed with a base or carrier oil such as sweet almond or grapeseed oil. The oils are usually used for massage treatments but can also be added to baths, or heated in water or in an oil-burner. Some oils have certain contra-indications for pregnancy and other conditions, so treatment should only be carried out by a qualified practitioner.

Bach Flower Remedies

Bach Flower Remedies is an holistic therapy developed by Dr Edward Bach in the 1920s and 1930s. He discovered 38 flowers that can help people to resolve both emotional and energetic imbalances. The remedies made from the flowers work in a gentle, healing way that is based on the idea that our diseases are caused by an imbalance between our body, soul and spirit. This therapy has been used for more than 70 years and is recommended by the World Health Organisation.

Counselling

Many healthy people seek a counsellor on a short- or long-term basis when they are coping with a particular problem, which can be either a crisis or a long-term situation they have finally decided to confront. A counsellor may work with couples or with an individual over many months or as little as four to six sessions. It is important to feel a rapport with the counsellor and if this is not the case then it is best to seek another person. Counselling can be offered free of charge through some GP's surgeries, or a GP can recommend a qualified practitioner.

Cranial/sacral osteopathy

Cranial osteopathy, also called craniosacral therapy, is a gentle manual treatment that aims to restore normal movement of the body and thus allow healthy function and integration of all body systems. This is a very subtle manipulation of the bones of the skull and sacral area of the back. When the body is subjected to trauma such as birth or injury, the flow of the cerebro-spinal fluid within the brain and spine can be disturbed or compromised. This is highly skilled work and is immensely helpful to clients from tiny babies to the elderly and infirm. The treatment helps to re-establish the body's own self-healing and self-regulating ability.

Deep tissue massage

Massage is one of the oldest healing therapies and records show it goes back thousands of years. In the fifth century, Hippocrates, the father of medicine wrote, 'The way to health is to have a scented bath and oiled massage every day.' Massage is most commonly used for relaxation and helps people with circulation problems, high blood pressure and heart disorders. The aim is to physically improve the cardiovascular, muscular and nervous systems. A massage will also stimulate the lymphatic system, which will help the body detoxify.

Remedial massage is more medically based and the practitioners are often also trained in physiotherapy. The massage is aimed at releasing stiffness in joints and muscles, making the body more supple and giving pain relief. Treatment is suitable for all age groups. A full case history is taken before a treatment plan is considered.

Herbalism

Herbs have been used for medicinal as well as culinary purposes for as long as humans have been on this planet. The World Health Organisation estimates that herbalism is three or more times more commonly practised than conventional medicine worldwide. It is estimated that 15 per cent of prescription medication is actually plant-based. In recent years herbal medicine has grown in popularity and medical herbalists are now an accepted part of the scientific community. Herbalism is aimed at treating the individual, and many herbalists mix up their own prescriptions of herbs, which may change as the client presents different symptoms on subsequent visits.

Homeopathy

Homeopaths boost the body's own healing ability by treating the whole person. They do not consider illness to be specific to the condition presented but instead see it as much more indicative of a sign of inner disharmony or imbalance. A

German physician, Samuel Hahnemann, first proposed this like-cures-like therapy in 1810. This is a similar notion to the theory behind vaccination but homeopathic doses are sub-atomically small in many cases – in others words the remedies given by a homeopath are extremely diluted, and the more diluted the dose, the greater the effect. Everyone including babies, animals and the chronically sick on medication can benefit from homeopathy. It is available from the British National Health Service and in several NHS homeopathic hospitals, and is practised by some GPs. There are also very able homeopaths who are not medically qualified but have a recognised qualification in homeopathy. Homeopathic preparations are readily available in pharmacies and health stores. All general, non-prescribed remedies are best taken in potency 6, which means one tablet, three times daily. Avoid taking 15 minutes either side of food, drink or toothpaste.

Hypnotherapy

Some doctors as well as qualified laypersons are trained to practise hypnotherapy. Hypnotherapist and patient come together in a series of one-to-one sessions, working through various emotional problems in a safe professional environment.

Conscious self-hypnosis is just one of the four natural states of consciousness that you enter quite regularly every day. Subliminal persuasion has been in everyday use ever since sound recording was invented. Used constructively – as with conscious self-hypnosis techniques on tape – you can work with yourself to eliminate unconscious self-sabotage and self-limiting negativity. When listening to the tape you are always aware of your surroundings and can react or stop the tape at any time. Many topics are covered on tape such as fear of flying, release from stress, phobias, bed-wetting, stuttering, concentration problems, etc. I recommend tapes produced by Duncan McColl, an experienced analytical hypnotherapist, gestalt therapist, and behavioural and management science consultant.

Indian head massage

Indian head massage, which has been practised in India for over 3,000 years, is becoming increasingly popular in the West. The ancient techniques have been adapted to suit modern demands, enabling therapists to work in a wide variety of settings including clinics, airports, schools, offices, hospices, beauty salons and even music festivals.

It is accessible, no special equipment is needed, and it takes less than half an hour to complete. Depending on the situation and location, the massage can be performed with or without natural oils, so clients do not need to disrobe and the working day need not be interrupted for long. Clients are also taught self-help techniques to use at home.

Indian head massage works not only on the scalp, as the name suggests, but also on the face, shoulders, upper back and arms. It works simultaneously on a physical and psychological level, counteracting physical and mental tension or lethargy, and encouraging well-being and vitality. It is particularly effective for stress-related conditions such as disturbed sleep patterns, mild depression, anxiety states and tension headaches. It has also proved beneficial for sinusitis, eye strain, jaw ache, migraines and poor circulation. The caring, physical contact of massage encourages the release of feel-good endorphins, which counteract the stress hormones in the bloodstream and boost the immune system, helping to fight infection.

Naturopathy

Naturopathy means 'nature cure' and naturopaths offer a holistic approach to healing the body, with the premise that the major cause of disease is a breakdown of the normal balance of the body. To correct this, the naturopath will take into account all the physical, emotional and environmental factors in a person's life. Naturopaths undergo intensive training over four years and combine a number of therapies and therapeutic devices to bring about health and balance.

Nutrition

The function of a nutritionist is to help you analyse your diet and pick up any shortfalls in it. You need to provide your body with the nutrients you need in order to reach your full potential, enable you to function well, and guard against deficiencies that can lead to degenerative diseases as you age. As well as providing the body with optimum levels of the 45 or so nutrients that you need for good health through diet, and where necessary supplements, it is wise to keep anti-nutrients such as refined foods, caffeine, alcohol and additives to a minimum. Just taking in the correct nutrients is not enough; you also need to be able to digest and absorb them, so addressing any digestive problems is also important.

Osteopathy

Osteopathy treats the whole person through the body's largest system, which is its framework of bones, joints, muscles and ligaments. It is a form of manipulative therapy. Osteopathy involves the careful and specific application of a highly developed sense of touch in both the diagnosis and the treatment of mechanical problems affecting any part of the body. Osteopaths treat back and neck pain as well as migraines, headaches, rheumatism, arthritis, repetitive strain injury, joint injuries and accident trauma such as whiplash. Conditions associated with pregnancy and childbirth are also suitable for treatment. Osteopathy is one of the most widely used types of complementary medicine. The osteopathic instruction is an intensive, full-time medically based training of four years' duration.

Phytobiophysics

The core scientific concept of phytobiophysics is that it harnesses the vibrational energy of plants to release energy blocks in the human body. The Flower Formulas, tiny sugar pills containing traces of plant tincture formulas, are based on the science of phytobiophysics, which has been researched and documented over the past 20 years by Professor Dame Diana Mossop. Qualified practitioners prescribe Flower Formulas with the correct frequency, creating immediate action to remove the energy blocks and bring back into balance whatever physical, emotional, mental or spiritual disturbances are evident.

Psychotherapy

Psychotherapy is designed to help people suffering from symptoms that may include anxiety, tension, or obsessive or compulsive behaviour. It is also helpful for many people who feel they want to be freed from behavioural patterns of a lifetime. The psychotherapist's aim is to deal with long-standing difficulties and to help the client to break out of a pattern of destructive behaviour. A psychotherapist may not be medically trained, so cannot prescribe medication, but will have taken extensive training through a professional body and will have undergone psychotherapy themselves as a precondition of training.

Glossary of terms

Abdominal area – this is situated below the chest from which it is separated by the diaphragm. It contains the digestive organs and excretory organs, and is lined by a membrane called the peritoneum.

Acupuncture – an ancient Chinese therapy that treats the body by puncturing it with fine needles on specific *meridian* points to balance and heal by regulating the *life force*. It is the most widely known complementary therapy in the West and is increasingly being used in conventional medical practice.

Acute – a condition having rapid onset (the opposite of *chronic*).

Adrenalin – an important hormone secreted from the medulla (core) of the adrenal gland. It has widespread effects on the muscles, circulation and sugar metabolism.

Allergy – a sensitivity disorder where the body becomes hypersensitive to particular allergens which provoke specific symptoms when encountered. Different allergies affect different tissues and produce localised or widespread effects. These can range from respiratory problems from pollen or house dust, gastro-enteritis or skin irritation to potentially fatal shock.

Allopathic medicine – orthodox medical treatment of diseases by drugs, surgery, etc.

Ankle-band – the part of the ankle at the base of the leg.

Ankle-bracelet – the same area as the *ankle-band* but is sometimes used in this book to specifically identify the area where the Zonal Triggers are located.

Antibody – a defensive substance within the organisms of the body that reacts to the presence of disease or toxins.

Arthritis – a generic term for a chronic joint disease characterised by loss of joint cartilage. Rheumatoid arthritis is an autoimmune disease where the synovial membrane of a joint gradually becomes swollen and inflamed.

Calf – the thick fleshy part of the back of the leg below the knee.

Capillary – a minute blood vessel that connects arteries with the veins.

Caterpillar bites – a reflexology term used to describe the finger or thumb techniques used to precisely work the reflexes by inching the finger (bent at the first joint) across the reflexes in tiny bites so as not to miss any area of the foot or hand. It can also be known as caterpillar walking; see also *thumb* and *finger walking*.

Cervical – refers to seven vertebrae bones making up the neck region of the spine.

Chronic – a condition of long duration (the opposite of *acute*).

Collagen – a fibrous connective tissue containing protein.

Contraindication – means unsuitable and is an indication of when not to treat.

Cranial nerves – the twelve pairs of nerves that have their roots at the base of the brain and supply parts of the head.

Crib sheet – basic instructions in abbreviated form.

Diaphragm – plays an important part in the mechanism of breathing. It is a strong, thin dome-shaped muscle that separates the thoracic and abdominal cavities.

Diaphragm Rocking – the diaphragm is represented as a horizontal line that runs below the ball of the hand or foot. This gentle rocking movement, when properly applied, appears to prioritise conditions most in need of help and pumps energy and relaxation to specific parts of the body. Disruptive sleep patterns improve dramatically and it has proved extremely effective in breaking long-term patterns of ill health. Diaphragm Rocking, along with Zonal Triggers, is one of the two most important techniques in the VRT repertoire.

Digit – finger or toe.

Dorsal (adjective) – referring to the top of the hand or foot.

Dorsum (noun) – the top of the hand or foot (as opposed to the palm or sole).

Endocrine – refers to the hormonal system of the body. The endocrine or ductless glands control long-term changes in the body. They secrete minute quantities of their hormone directly into the body.

Endocrine Flush – the endocrine reflexes (or those of any system) are worked sequentially and simultaneously on both hands for greater effect. Each system of reflexes can also be worked one hand at a time combining nail-on-nail pressure with the pituitary reflex.

Fingertip Pressure – a powerful way of working all the weight-bearing fingers by exerting pressure on the fingertips.

Fingerpressure walking – a standard reflexology technique where the finger is bent at the first joint and *inches* across the foot or hand, minutely making contact with the reflexes. *Caterpillar walking* is also a term used to describe this technique.

Forefinger – the first finger after the thumb. Also known as the *index* finger.

Genitalia – the reproductive organs of the male and female, particularly the external parts such as the penis, testicles, labia and clitoris.

Glands – ductless vessels or structures that synthesise and secrete certain fluids for use in the body or for excretion.

Glucose – an important source of energy and one of the constituents of sucrose and starch which supply glucose after digestion. It is stored in the body in the form of *glycogen.*

Glycogen – can be readily broken down into glucose. It is stored in the muscles and liver and is the principal form in which carbohydrate is stored in the body.

Harmoniser – a technique to help stabilise the body and prevent any side effects. It can accelerate the healing processes.

Healing crisis – a natural reaction to a complementary treatment which can occasionally result when the body is stimulated to throw off toxins too quickly. This can result in a short period, usually a few hours, of possible vomiting or bowel disorders, skin sensitivity or increased pain. It can also result in a headache. All these symptoms can often be prevented by asking the client to drink much more water following a treatment and by applying the Harmoniser. Some practitioners have created a minor healing crisis for their clients by using VRT for up to 15 minutes in a treatment, instead of five, against all good advice. In all reports the patient felt better than ever once the symptoms subsided, but the discomfort suffered had been unnecessary. Side effects are a milder version of a healing crisis.

Helper reflexes – these specifically refer to the new reflexes discovered in VRT that support, and are linked, to the original reflexes, that is, the helper heart, ovary and diaphragm reflexes. By working the helper reflexes a treatment can be enhanced.

Holistic – an approach to health that aims to treat the person as an entity where the body, mind and spirit are assumed to co-exist and are all given consideration.

Homeostasis – a Greek word meaning a state of balance or equilibrium.

Hypertension – high blood pressure.

Hypotension – low blood pressure.

Immune system – a general term for a complex system that enables the body to resist infection and fight disease. This is afforded by the presence of circulating antibodies and white blood cells.

Index finger – the first finger after the thumb. Also known as the forefinger.

Knuckle Dusting – a means of working the dorsum (top) of the hand or foot with the knuckles. The fist of the hand uses light twisting and sweeping movements. It is extremely powerful in treating such diverse conditions as asthma, depression and Irritable Bowel Syndrome. Use for only 15 seconds on each hand.

Lateral – refers to the outside edge of the hand or foot.

Libido – the sexual drive. Usually refers to the degree of intensity.

Life force – an energy and innate form of self healing within the body.

Longitudinal zones – ten vertical reflexology zones in the body, five on each side and starting on the toes and fingers, that act as conduits for healing and stimulation from reflex points to particular parts of the body.

Lumbar – refers to the five lower vertebrae in the back. These are situated between the thoracic vertebrae and the sacrum/coccyx at the base of the spine. The lumbar spine refers to the lower back.

Lymph glands – principally found in the neck, groin and armpits. The small vessels that link them are called lymphatics; they contain a thin fluid called lymph.

Lymph – the thin fluid present within the lymphatic system. Lymph contains some protein and some cells which are mainly lymphocytes.

Lymphatic system – a network of vessels in the body that carries water, proteins, electrolytes, etc., in the form of lymph from the tissue fluids to the bloodstream.

ME (Myalgic encephalitis) – a form of post-viral syndrome often following influenza or glandular fever. It has many symptoms, including chronic tiredness, digestive problems and general lack of energy. Post-viral conditions are usually identified as ME when the patient presents painful, tender muscles. The condition can last for years.

Medial – refers to the inside edge of the foot or hand.

Meridian Lines – a term in acupuncture that describes the channels that run through the body carrying the *life force* or chi. There are 14 main meridians in Chinese acupuncture that run from the hands and feet to the body and the head.

Metabolism – the collection of all the chemical and physical changes that take place within the body. It is the process by which the body grows and functions.

Metacarpals – the longest bones in the hands. They connect to phalanges (finger bones).

Metatarsals – the longest bones in the feet. They connect to the phalanges (toe bones).

Nail-working – a powerful technique by which the sensitive reflexes on the nails are stimulated by the pressure of the reflexologist's nail on a defined grid-system.

Nerve/neural pathways – denote the complex system of 31 pairs of spinal nerves that emanate from the spinal cord to various parts of the body and relay messages to and from the brain.

Nervous system *(Autonomic)* – supplies all the body structures over which we have no control. It is divided into two separate parts – the sympathetic and parasympathetic systems.

Neural pathway reflexes – are situated in the same area as the primary set of spinal reflexes which run down the lateral and medial edges of the foot and hand (inside edge). The term *neural pathways* refers to the 31 pairs of nerves which emanate from the central nervous system to various parts of the body and relay messages to and from the brain. The *spinal cord* is protected by the vertebrae that make up the spinal column.

Oedema – excessive accumulation of fluid in the body tissues. Subcutaneous oedema commonly occurs in the legs and ankles. Reflexologists should work very gently on swollen feet or work the hands instead.

Orthopaedic – preventative and corrective treatment of the skeletal system.

Osteopathy – a gentle manipulation of the muscular-skeletal system to realign the framework of the body so that it interacts efficiently with the nervous, circulatory and other systems.

Palmar Pressure technique – pressure is only placed on the ball of the hand and fingers so the weight-bearing palm reflexes can be worked as well.

Palming – a gentle technique where the heel of the palm is applied to the dorsum of the foot in firm pressing and sweeping movements.

Phalanges – the finger and toe bones.

Pituitary gland – the master gland of the endocrine system, a pea-sized body attached to the hypothalamus at the base of the skull. It controls the function of all other glands in the body.

Pituitary Pinch – this is a very powerful VRT technique where the pituitary reflexes (the master gland of the endocrine system) on the thumbs and big toes are simultaneously stimulated when the client is weight-bearing.

Plantar – the sole of the foot.

Points – in this book it is simply another word for *reflexes.*

Post-viral syndrome – often follows influenza or glandular fever. There are many symptoms including chronic tiredness, digestive problems and a general lack of energy. Post-viral conditions are usually identified as *ME (Myalgic encephalitis)* only when a patient presents painful, tender muscles and the condition has been present for many months.

Premenstrual tension – a collection of symptoms including bloating, depression, irritability and inability to concentrate that usually occur during the week preceding menstruation.

Referral areas – are useful as an extra tool in reflexology when you want to treat, for example, a painful right ankle. You would work the right wrist instead. The basic rule is as follows: always link limbs on the same side of the body, that is, right to right. *Hip* links with *shoulder, thigh* links with *upper arm, elbow* links with *knee, calf* links with *forearm, ankle* links with *wrist* and *hand* links with *foot.*

Referred pain – a pain in the body in an area other than the source. This occurs because the sensory nerves share common pathways to the spinal cord and the brain.

Reflexes – sensitive minute *points* on the feet that are connected to specific parts of the body and can sometimes feel quite tender if they correspond to a malfunctioning part of the body. However, painful areas of the feet do not always indicate ill health, they can simply show vitality! Reflexes can also become tender due to a physical problem on the foot itself that is totally unconnected with reflexology, and you must be aware of this possibility when treating clients. A reflexologist is trained to detect the difference – but the golden rule for everyone is to ease off a painful reflex and work it more gently.

Reflexology – an ancient natural therapy that describes a healing energy that flows from hundreds of specific reflexes in the feet. These reflexes correspond to all the organs, glands and parts of the skeletal system in the body. By gently stimulating certain points with fingers and thumbs, the body itself responds to bring about self-healing and *homeostasis* (the Greek word for 'balance').

Rotating movement – refers to a standard reflexology technique where the finger or thumb is placed firmly on a reflex point and rotated in small, circular movements to stimulate an energetic response in a particular part of the body.

Sciatic nerve – the major nerve in the leg, which runs from the lower end of the spine down the leg to below the thigh.

Sebaceous glands – open into the hair follicles. They are simple or branched glands in the skin that secrete an oily substance called sebum.

Self-help VRT techniques – essential to the well-being of all therapists and carers: a form of instant first aid that can be applied anywhere. The synergistic approach to self-help is very powerful and you can even work your own foot and hand at the same time.

Senses – sight, hearing, smell, taste and touch are the faculties through which the external world is appreciated.

Side-effects – in the context of complementary therapies, side-effects are mild natural reactions to a treatment which can occasionally result when the body is stimulated to throw off toxins, unlike a *healing crisis*, which is a stronger reaction.

Spinal cord – supplies 31 pairs of extremely complex nerves that branch off along the spinal cord to various parts of the body. Reflexologists refer to these in a simplified form when working the *neural pathway reflexes.*

Steroid – a group of organic hormones that include male and female sex hormones plus the hormones of the adrenal cortex.

Synergistic – combined or coordinated actions that, when used together, increase the effect of the other. In VRT the simultaneous working of the hand and foot reflexes greatly increases the response of the body as opposed to working each reflex separately.

Synergistic reflexology – a technique where hand and foot reflexes are worked simultaneously. This technique can accelerate the body's response and, in orthopaedic cases, increased mobility has sometimes been achieved in minutes. Synergistic reflexology also works when the client is lying or sitting down, and the person being treated can be taught to work their own appropriate hand reflexes.

Systems of the body – these comprise various groups of organs, glands, nerves and skeletal structures, each of which performs a specific function. The systems of the body are interdependent.

Tendon – a tough band of fibrous tissue forming the end of a muscle and attached to the bone. Reflexologists should take care not to exert undue pressure on the tendon on the medial (inside) palm of the hand or sole of the foot. No pressure at all should be placed on the tendon when the hand or foot is weight-bearing, as in Plantar Stepping and Metacarpal Pressure.

Thigh – the upper part of the leg between the hip and the knee.

Thoracic – refers to 12 bones of the backbone or spine to which the ribs are attached. They are situated between the *cervical* and *lumbar* vertebrae.

Thumb pressure walking – a standard reflexology technique where the thumb is bent at the first joint and inches across the foot or hand minutely making contact with the reflexes. The term *caterpillar bites* is also sometimes used to describe this technique.

Toxin – a poison produced by living organisms in the body, especially bacteria.

Transverse zones – horizontal lines on the foot that mark the shoulder girdle, waistline and pelvic floor position and the relative position of the corresponding reflexes on the hands and feet.

Varicose veins – these can be fine or thick veins that are distorted, lengthened and tortuous. The most common site is in the legs.

Vertebra (plural vertebrae) – one of the 33 bones that comprise the spine or backbone. The arch of each vertebra contains part of the spinal cord. Vertebrae are bound together by ligaments and intervertebral discs.

Vertical Reflex Therapy – the overall term for the form of reflexology that treats the dorsum (top) of the hand or foot. These reflexes become far more sensitive and responsive to pressure when weight-bearing.

Whole Body Brush – the knuckles or fingertips are used to work around the wrist Zonal Triggers and the dorsum is brushed and pinched from the wrist to the fingertips.

Zonal Triggers – deep reflex points on the ankles that appear to accelerate the healing to deep-seated problems in the body when linked to two specific reflexes. They are simple to detect and use and are, along with Diaphragm Rocking, one of the two most important techniques in the VRT repertoire.

Zones – ten longitudinal energetic reflexology lines which run throughout the body starting at the fingers and the toes, with five on each side. The flow of energy affects and stimulates all parts of the body situated within each zone. Reflexology acts as a stimulus to remove blocks in the zones that can create ill-health and inhibit the life force.

Useful addresses

Reflexology training addresses

Booth VRT Ltd
Suite 205
60 Westbury Hill
Westbury-on-Trym
Bristol BS9 3UJ
Tel: 01179 626746
Email: contact@boothvrt.com
www.boothvrt.com

Vertical Reflex Therapy courses are run for qualified reflexologists throughout the UK and internationally by Lynne Booth and VRT appointed tutors. For details about VRT, course venue information and telephone numbers of trained VRT practitioners in specific areas, send a stamped addressed envelope to the above address stating your requirement.

Advanced Reflexology Training (ART)
Anthony Porter, Director
Hollyfield Avenue
London N11 3BY
Tel: 020 8368 0865
Fax: 020 8368 1269
Email: artreflex@btinternet.com
www:artreflex.com

ART courses are run in the UK and internationally for qualified reflexologists.

Association of Reflexologists
Old Gloucester Street
London, WC1N 3XX
Tel: 0870 5673320
Email:aor@assocmanagement.co.uk
www.aor.org.uk

The Association is the largest UK independent reflexology organisation and aims to maintain high standards of practice.

International Council of Reflexologists
PO Box 78060,
Westcliffe Postal Outlet,
Hamilton,
Ontario L9C 7N5,
Canada
Tel: +1 905 387 8449
Email: icr@mountaincable.net

International Institute of Reflexology
Head Office (UK)
Hill House
255 Turleigh
Bradford-on-Avon
Wiltshire BA15 2HG
Tel/Fax: 01225 865899
Email:reflexology_uk@hotmail.com
www.reflexology_uk.co.uk

International Institute of Reflexology
International Head Office
PO Box 12642
St Petersburg, FL

33733–2642 USA
Tel: 001 727 343 4811
Email: ftreflex@concentric.net
www.reflexology-usa.net

The Institute's professional courses, accredited by the Open and Distance Learning Quality Control Council, are taught throughout the world.

Kristine Walker Hand Reflexology
223 Hartington Road
Brighton
East Sussex BN2 3PA
Email:walkerkristine@hotmail.com

Kristine Walker has greatly influenced hand reflexology teaching and her book *Hand Reflexology* is also a very useful reference text when using VRT synergistically.

Manual Neuro-Therapy and
Neuro-Reflexology
Nico Pauly
IRSK-WINGS
Oude Veurnestraat 75 C
8900 Ieper, Belgium
Tel: 00 32 57 33.60.83
Fax: 00 32 57 33.50.65
Email: irsk-wings@itinera.be

New Zealand Reflexology
Association
PO Box 31084
Auckland 9
New Zealand
Tel: + 64 9 486 1918

Reflexology Association of
America
K-Box PMB#585, 2059
4012 S Rainbow Boulevard,
Las Vegas,
Nevada 89103-2
USA
Email: inforaa@reflexology-
usa.org
www.reflexology-usa.org

Reflexology Association of
Australia
RAA - National Enquiries
PO Box 366,
Cammeray
NSW 2062
Australia
Tel: + 0500 502 250
www.reflexology.org.au

Reflexology Association of
Canada
P.O. Box 83008
Edmonton
Alberta T5T 6S1
Canada
Tel: + 780-443-4246
Email:
adminserv@reflexologycanada.ca
www.reflexologycanada.ca

Reflexology in Europe Network
(R.I.E.N.)
Bovenover 59
1025 JJ Amsterdam
The Netherlands
Tel/Fax: 31 20 636 3915
Email: h.van.der.werff@freeler.nl
www.reflexeurope.org

The School of Precision
Reflexology
38 South Street
Exeter
Devon EX1 1ED
Tel: 01392 499360
Fax: 01392 410954
Email: jan.sch@breathemail.net
www.schoolofcomplementaryh
ealth.co.uk

The South African Reflexology
Society
PO Box 1780
New Germany, 3620
South Africa
Tel/Fax: + 27 31 7028531
Email:admin@sareflexology.
org.za
www.sareflexology.org.za

Other relevant addresses

Following are contact details of
organisations that can offer
advice on therapies
complementary to reflexology.

Acupuncture
British Acupuncture Council
63 Jeddo Road
London W12 9HQ
Tel: 020 8735 0400
Email: info@acupuncture.org.uk
www.acupuncture.org.uk

Alexander Technique
British Society of Teachers of
the Alexander Technique
129 Camden Mews
London NW1 9AH
Tel: 020 7284 3338
Email: david@stat.org.uk
www.stat.org.uk

Applied Kinesiology
The Wessex School of
Kinesiology
321 Nore Road
Portishead
Bristol BS20 8EN
Tel/Fax: 01275 846683
Email:pauline.noakes@lineone.
net

Aromatherapy
Aromatherapy & Allied
Practitioners' Association
8 George Street
Croydon CRO 1PA
Tel/Fax: 020 8680 7761
Email: aromatherapyuk@aol.com

Bach Flower Remedies
The Dr Edward Bach Centre
Mount Vernon
Sotwell
Wallingford
Oxon OX10 OPZ
Tel: 01471 834678
www.bachcentre.com

Counselling
British Association for
Counselling and Psychotherapy
1 Regent Place
Rugby
Warwickshire CV21 2PJ
Tel: 0870 4435252
Email: bacp@bacp.co.uk
www.bacp.co.uk

Deep Tissue Massage
APNT (Association of Physical
and Natural Therapists)
27 Old Gloucester Street
London WC1N 3XX
Tel: 07966 181588
Email: apntsource@lineone.net
www.apnt.org.uk

Herbalism
The Herb Society
Sulgrave Manor
Sulgrave
Banbury
Oxfordshire OX17 2SD
Tel: 01295 768899
Fax: 01295 768069
Email: info@herbsociety.co.uk
www.herbsociety.co.uk

Homeopathy
Homeopathic Medical
Association
6 Livingstone Road
Gravesend
Kent DA12 5DZ
Tel: 01474 560336
Email: info@the-hma.org

The Society of Homeopaths
4a Artisan Road
Northampton NN1 4HU
Tel: 01604 621400
Fax: 01604 622622
Email: info@homeopathy-soh.org

Hypnotherapy
The Hypnotherapy Association
14 Crown Street
Chorley
Lancashire PR7 1DX
Tel: 01257 262124
Email: bha@lineone.net
www.zednet.co.uk/bhahypno
therapy

Pilgrim Tapes
PO Box 107
Shrewsbury
Shropshire SY1 1ZZ
Tel: 01743 821270

Indian Head Massage
The London Centre of Indian
Champissage
136 Holloway Road
London N7 8DD
Tel: 020 7609 3590
Fax: 020 7607 4228

Email:indianchampissage@
yahoo.com
www.indianchampissage.com

Naturopathy
The British Naturopathic
Association
Goswell House
2 Goswell Road
Street
Somerset BA16 0JG
Tel: 0870 7456 984
Email: admin@naturopaths.
org.uk
www.naturopaths.org.uk

British Naturopathic and
Osteopathic Association
6 Netherall Gardens
London NW3 5RR
Tel: 020 7435 7830
www.bcno.ac.uk

Nutrition
Institute for Optimum Nutrition
Blades Court
Deodar Road
London SW15 2NU
Tel: 020 8877 9993
Email: info@ion.ac.uk
www.ion.ac.uk

Osteopathy
General Osteopathic Council
Osteopathy House
176 Tower Bridge Road
London SE1 3LU
Tel: 020 7357 6655
Email: info@osteopathy.org.uk
www.osteopathy.org.uk

Phytobiotics
The Institute of
Phytobiophysics
D&P Ltd
10 St James Street
St Helier
Jersey JE2 3QZ
Tel: 01534 738737
Fax 01534 618756
www.phytobiophysics.co.uk

Psychotherapy
United Kingdom Council for
Psychotherapy
167–169 Great Portland Street
London W1W 5PF
Tel: 020 7436 3002
Fax: 020 7436 3013
Email: ukcp@psychotherapy.
org.uk
www.psychotherapy.org.uk

Recommended Reading

Atkinson, Mary, *The Art of Indian Head Massage*, Carlton Books, 2000
Booth, Lynne, *Vertical Reflexology*, Piatkus Books, 2000
Goodman, Dr Sandra, *Nutrition and Cancer: State of the Art*, Positive Health Publications Ltd, 1998
Houghton, Paul, *A Guide to Homeopathic Remedies*, Souvenir Press, 2001
Kavounas, Alice, *Water – Pure Therapy*, Kyle Cathie Ltd, 2000
Kenton, Leslie, *Ten Steps to a Natural Menopause*, Vermillion, 1999
Marsden, Kathryn, *The Complete Book of Food Combining*, Piatkus Books, 2000
Norman, Laura, *The Reflexology Handbook*, Piatkus Books, 1989
Van Straten, Michael, *The Good Health Directory*, Newleaf, 2000
Walker, Kristine, *Hand Reflexology – A Student's Guide*, Quay Books, 2001
Wills, Judith, *The Food Bible*, Quadrille, 1998

Monthly publications
Positive Health, by subscription (tel: 0117 983 8851) or from newsagents/health shops.
What Doctors Don't Tell You, by subscription (tel: 020 8944 9555).

Index

pineal gland 118, 150
pineal reflex 80
pituitary gland 118, 150
Pituitary Pinch 41, 56, 73, 104, 106, 166
pituitary reflexes 21, 79–85, 91, 111
Porter, Anthony 6, 17
posture 7, 34, 51, 57, 123, 175
pregnancy 9, 172
priority conditions, addressing 168
prostate gland 146, 161, 162–3
    see also uterus/prostate reflex
psychotherapy 141, 149, 185

referral reflexes 52
reflexes
    differences between hand/feet 24
    tender 4, 9, 15, 19, 32, 98
    see also specific reflexes
relaxation techniques 13–15, 94–5
repetitive strain injury 177–8
reproductive problems 162–4, 172
reproductive reflexes 162, 163
reproductive system 115, 160–4
respiratory reflexes 136
respiratory system 115, 134–7
response times 72
right lymphatic duct 130
Riley, Joe Shelby 2

sacral nerves 118
Secondary nail technique 75, 84, 85–7
self-help 33, 92–112, 168, 176
    client doubts regarding 179
    conventional reflexology for 93, 94–100
    frequency of treatments 43, 73
    introduction to the techniques 93–4
    nail-working for 78, 79, 110–11
    for specific conditions 116, 120–1, 125,
        129, 133, 137, 141, 145, 148, 154,
        159, 164
    synergistic reflexology on passive
        hands 93, 94, 100–4
    types 93
    weight-bearing VRT and synergistic
        reflexology 92, 93, 94, 104–6
self-hypnosis 121, 145, 182
sense organ reflexes 157, 158
sense organs 115, 155–9
shoulder problems 63, 123, 172, 177–8

shoulder reflexes 49–51, 86
skeletal charts, hand/foot 46
skeletal problems x, 122–5
skeletal reflexes 123, 124
skeletal system 114, 122–5
skin 155–6
solar plexus reflex 42, 54, 100, 107
sperm 161
spinal nerves 117–18
spinal reflexes 17, 36–8, 57
    squeezing 95
    twisting 14
    working in self-help treatments 102,
        111
spine/spinal cord 33, 59–61, 88, 122
spleen 130, 131
sports therapy 70, 127–9
stomach reflexes 98, 99
stress xii, 153–4, 172, 174
strokes 59, 139–41, 173
surroundings 57, 175
sweat glands 155
synergistic reflexology 44–5, 52–3
    in basic VRT 166
    combinations 73
    in complete hand VRT 71–2
    definition 104, 166
    guidelines 56
    method 45
    positions for 35, 44, 48
    use in self-help treatments 93, 94,
        101–4, 104–6
    therapists' posture for 51
    and Zonal Trigger reflexes 48, 49–51,
        57

tapping nail-on-nail technique 78
taste buds 156
tendons 126–7
testes 152, 160, 161
    see also ovary/testes helper reflex;
        ovary/testes reflex
thalamus 118
therapists
    investigating 9, 180
    posture of 7, 34, 51, 57
thoracic calf reflexes
    on the arms 32
    on the legs 31
thoracic duct 130